# The
# GALL BLADDER
## Survival Guide

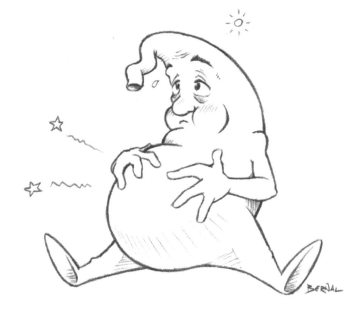

How to live a normal life with a dysfunctional or missing Gall Bladder.

## Written and illustrated by J. Bernal

1

*I dedicate this book to Mom:*

Thanks for those stomach-churning medical gross-out
stories over the dinner table when we were kids.

# Table of Contents

# 1: Introduction

A shocking 750,000 gall bladders are removed every year, just in the United States of America. Few of the patients of this procedure, if any, are given proper instructions on what to do afterwards. They are typically told to go home and continue life as normal, and to consider cutting back on their fat intake.

If you are reading this, chances are that you already know you were given bad advice. It's easy to understand why: surgeons are not nutritionists. They spend years specializing in a task learning how to remove a compromised or gangrenous organ without harming the patient.

You wouldn't want a surgeon operating on you who spent half as much time cutting bodies because he spent the other half studying digestive balance, just as when you consult a nutritionist you want to make sure they spent their time studying proper nutrition and not removing organs with a scalpel or scope. Those people cutting out your organs and telling you how to take care of yourself afterwards probably still have their gall bladders.

It would be nice if they teamed up, but the reality is that it is not practical. After all, providing you came through the procedure with flying colors, so what if you have diarrhea, or you are getting depressed, or your sex drive and performance have taken a dive? There are drugs for that, right? Be happy that you are not dead!

You already have enough crap to deal with in your life, literally and figuratively. Let me save you some time, money, and frustration.

This book will help supply you with proper knowledge based on real science and experience from real people who have gone through it, experienced the reality of the nutritional side effects, and have triumphed over them.

It is written primarily for you who have had your gall bladder removed. It may also be helpful to you who suffer from gallstones or generally uncooperative gall bladders, and are considering surgery or other treatments.

While by all means not a comletely exhaustive compendium of digestive biochemistry, this book should provide you fairly good coverage of all things gall bladder related. Nothing here is secret knowledge, and most can be found for free on the internet; I am just trying to save you time and torment by filtering out the garbage, compiling everything in one place, and explaining how your guts work in simple and understandable terms so as to aid your return to normal bowel function. I suffered long enough looking for answers; now you don't have to repeat my misery.

Some rare souls do not experience any noticeable problems after their gall bladders have been removed. I am not one of those lucky ones. If you are reading this, you are likely equally unlucky, and you want to know what to do to fix things.

**There *is* hope-- read on!**

I lost my gall bladder in 2006. Yes, lost. As in "had I been presented with any possibility of keeping it, I would have done so."

I searched for many years in vain for the source of knowledge that would return my digestion to normal. None exists, until now. Which, frankly, is fascinating considering the number of people who are surgically separated from their gall bladders every year.

Granted the side-effects of a missing gall bladder are not immediately lethal, and "grumpy" bowels are semi-tolerable, but life does not need to be that way. You CAN improve things, with the proper knowledge and a little bit of effort spent getting to know your new digestive system.

Not a single one of the gall-bladder-less people I have met in my research were given proper nutritional information, counseling, not even the slightest of warnings from their doctors about the inevitable and ongoing post-surgery symptoms.

The doctor who removed my gall bladder told me I didn't have to make any adjustments to my diet. Was he ever wrong! Well, I didn't *have* to make changes to my diet, but I wouldn't like the results either: vitamin deficiencies, chronic and urgent diarrhea, gas, bloating...

The fact of the matter is that you *will* have to make some adjustments, because without your gall bladder, no matter how healthy you think you eat, you are not getting the proper digestion and nutrition you need. I am not a doctor, but you do not need to be one to understand this stuff.

The good news is that the nutritional deficiencies and bowel-related unpleasantness are easy to counteract through diet, affordable over-the-counter nutritional supplements, and/or non-drug prescription dietary additives, which makes the lack of doctor-patient information/support all the more shocking and frustrating.

This book is an attempt to fill the informational void-- what works, what doesn't, the chemistry behind it all (broken down in layman's terms) and how to properly compensate for your new underachieving digestive system.

Since all things in the gall bladder world result in digestion (or not-quite-digestion), we will spend some time discussing our excrement. There's just not an easy way to do this without sounding like a stuffy academic, so I shall attempt to make it humorous. This should not only break the ice, but help you remember key points in the gall bladder function, proper digestion and nutrient absorption, what we need to do now to ensure good nutrition and manufacture of high-quality poop that you will be proud of once more.

# 2: Losing Big in Vegas

April 2006: Las Vegas, Nevada: My wife and I were in Las Vegas on vacation. She was there for a trade show; I was there to visit my friend Todd and partake in the gambling, shows, restaurants, and general gluttony for which the city is famous.

Actually, before I get to the gluttony and its resulting horror, let's rewind a week.

...

Late March 2006: St. Augustine, Florida. After eating a particularly greasy hot dog for lunch, I was doubled over by extreme pain in my abdomen. My wife and I were in the car. Fortunately I was not driving.

Having passed kidney stones before, I thought that this might be another one. Knowing full well that there is nothing that can be done but wait in extreme pain until a kidney stone passes, I was inclined to take loads of painkillers, drink loads of water, and try to spend loads of time unconscious until it was done ruining my day.

The pain didn't abate. It continued to get worse and worse. I was sweating, shaking, and vomiting uncontrollably. No matter what position I tried contorting my body into: standing, sitting, curled this way and that, the pain would not go away. There was no comfortable position to be had. I asked my wife to take me to the hospital.

The hospital part is kind of hazy, as I was either

blacking out from the pain or blocking the traumatic experience from my brain, but after an unknown wait in the ER writhing in my seat and making periodic sprints to the trash can to puke, the doctors were ready to see me.

They took my temperature, blood pressure, x-rays of my abdomen, gave me prescriptions for a strong painkiller and an anti-nausea medication, told me I had stomach flu, and that it would pass in a few days if I went home. Thank you, bye-bye, next!

Meanwhile an incredibly evil gallstone 1.4 centimeters in diameter (the size of my thumb) was blocking my bile duct, and my gall bladder was turning gangrenous...

...

Back in Vegas: Feeling perfectly fine, thinking it was just some stomach bug from that Satanic hot dog, I went on with my life as if nothing was wrong with me. That is, until I ate a big buffet dinner at one of the casino hotels...

Back at Todd's house, the pain started. At first I tried to be discreet about it, as people tend to worry when they hear labored gagging sounds coming from their guest bathroom. However, after watching my ghost-pale zombified corpse pacing the house, pausing periodically to bend over and clutch its gut, wipe the sweat from its face, and then scramble quickly to the bathroom to offer another set of painful dry heaves into the toilet, the folks present asked politely if, just maybe, they should take me to the hospital.

Once again the hospital part is a bit unclear. I

9

remember sitting in the waiting room for what seemed like an eternity. At this point I was too weak to keep vomiting, so I just kind of leaned around to either side, front, back, whatever position was least horrible in the chair. I remember the hospital people propping me back up in the chair a few times and checking my pulse, probably because I passed out and fell onto the waiting room floor.

Then I was on a gurney and they were asking me the usual triage questions, gathering name and address information, etc. I kept telling them to check my wallet. I didn't want to talk to them; that required remaining conscious, and anything but unconsciousness at that point in time was not ideal.

Eventually the morphine drip washed through me and my brain could function again, sort of. They asked my permission for an ultrasound. "Do whatever you have to do, just fix it," was my response.

...

Let's rewind a bit more, not to a specific time but to what was going on over the previous year or so. While my gall bladder was undergoing what can best be described as "gradual decline", there were definite symptoms, which I did not know the cause of, and thought would eventually go away.

To put it bluntly, my poop had gone from regular and firm to completely soft-serve. I had gas that I can only describe as being so foul as to peel paint from walls. Not just in concentration but in volume. When you start to offend yourself, it is time to see a doctor. I should have, but I didn't. It will go away, right? Probably just something I ate. I really should start eating more healthy things...

To top off the disgusting symptoms, my bowels became so erratic and uncontrollable that I could hardly go anywhere in public without difficulty. Constantly irritable bowels coupled with bile leaking whenever it wanted to... well, it was gross. Being a stubborn idiot I kept the suffering to myself and didn't dare tell my wife I was having problems; the stench of my gas was becoming a big enough strain on our marriage.

A couple of months before the Vegas incident I went camping/hiking with my mother and brothers in the Oregon wilderness. I was so gassed up from something I ate, and my bowels were so irritated, that I spent most of my time in bed. You don't want to go hiking in the mountains when the next strenuous step could mean you will crap your pants. Granted you are in the wilderness with only your family, but who wants to hike miles back to camp in crapped pants? I can't imagine how horrible it was for them at night, stuck in the cabin with my toxic gas cloud.

I reached my "I can't take this anymore" moment shortly before St. Augustine and Las Vegas. But it will go away eventually; it has to, right?

...

Back in Vegas: A doctor woke me up to tell me that during the ultrasound they found a very large gallstone blocking my bile duct, there was evidence of gangrene, and that the whole thing had to go: stone, bladder, and all. Yes, sir, if you do not remove it in short order, you will be dead within 48 hours. Those words don't hold quite the gravity they should when you are high on morphine.

I don't remember the ultrasound. I do remember asking him if there was any way to save my gall bladder, but he explained that considering my history and what they saw in the ultrasound, it was no doubt very badly infected and was not going to be salvageable. I must have told them about St Augustine at some point during my triage interrogation. He had some nice color pictures of gall bladders and gall stones and tried explaining the procedure to remove it, but my eyes were rolling back in my skull and I had more interest in going back to painless, morphine-induced sleep.

In and out of consciousness again, different rooms, different halls, someone asks me to sign a form allowing the surgery and I do. It felt like a week had passed. Then they wheeled me into a room where they shaved by belly, put a gas mask on me, and asked me to count to ten. I think I made it to three.

I woke up during the procedure and reached forward to pull the curtain away, asking them if I could watch, "I wanna see!" The anesthesiologist quickly turned up the gas and I was again whisked away to happy-land.

When I woke up my arms were strapped to the gurney. My belligerent curiosity must have spooked the folks in the ER. When the doctor came by to take the cuffs off of me, he told me that my gall bladder was definitely gangrenous and there was no way they could have saved it. As a result I would need to be loaded full of antibiotics and observed for another 24 hours minimum. (otherwise, with modern laparoscopic surgery, gall bladder removals are an outpatient procedure)

Still in a drugged haze, I demanded to see my gall bladder. Unfortunately, it had already been sent off to the lab for testing. I was disappointed; after all this pain and suffering I wanted to see the culprit face to face. And maybe keep it in a prison of glass and formaldehyde on my shelf, a trophy of sorts. It made sense at the time.

After my 24 hours of observation was over I was released. They wanted to keep me longer but I was drugged, in pain, extremely abrasive, and demanded to go home. They reluctantly let me leave after I could prove I was mobile enough to walk around the recovery ward.

My first post-surgery poop was the first, most solid, perfect poop I would create in a long time, and the last, most solid, perfect poop I would create in a long time.

It would be years of trial and error, and many urgent runs to the toilet before I got straightened out. Even to this day I am not 100% perfect but I am a lot better than when I started out.


I haven't been back to Las Vegas since.

# 3: It's Gone! Now What?

When your gall bladder is gone, either literally or figuratively, most of us are told to go about our business as normal. Some of us are lucky enough that we feel no immediate side effects nor changes in our digestion. However many of us will quickly notice things are not normal.

Some of us are told to eat a low-fat diet. This is absolutely, positively 100% backwards. With your gall bladder missing, your body will already be hungry for the fats it needs; holding back on your fats is like cutting off your nose to spite your face.

The first short-term thing you will probably notice is soft stool. Your bowels will likely be irritable and rapid. You may be gassier than normal, and experience times of extreme bloating. You may experience regular diarrhea. You may experience uncontrollable leakage for a while. In general, your butt will probably become your least-favorite body part, and it will be spending a lot of time getting to know the toilet.

### Step 1: The New Black.
Throw out all of your white underwear and buy new replacements in black. If you were suffering from gall bladder failure before your operation, you will understand why. You're going to be having a rough enough time adjusting to your new digestive process; spare yourself the embarrassment of having racing stripes in your undies.

### *Step 2: Get checked for Coeliac Disease.*

Coeliac Disease is an autoimmune disease triggered by proteins in wheat products. Not all gall bladder patients will have Coeliac Disease, but many Coeliac Disease patients will eventually become gall bladder patients.

After experiencing gall bladder failure, you will definitely want to know whether or not you have Coeliac Disease so you know how to drive your new digestive system and keep it from crashing out of control. Getting tested is as easy as checking blood samples for specific antibodies. For more information on this disease and what it does, see page 63, "The Coeliac Connection."

The silver lining to the Coeliac Disease cloud is that the damage can be reversed by following a gluten-free diet. It won't grow you a new gall bladder but it will wake up a sleepy one if it's still around.

### *Step 3: Get a Heidelberg Capsule test.*

The gall bladder isn't the only part that could have issues-- your stomach acid levels could also be to blame. Bile and stomach acid go hand in hand-- bile helps deactivate the acidity of your stomach contents. If the balance is off, you will have problems down the line in your digestive tract.

The Heidelberg Capsule is a tiny radio transmitter which you swallow. As it passes through your digestive tract, it broadcasts measured levels of pH (acidity).

After this test, your doctor can explain to you whether or not your stomach acid levels are correct, and if your biliary system and digestive tract are responding adequately to the acidity. With this information in hand, you will know your guts better, and in turn be able to calculate whether or not you need to...

### *Step 4: Buy or order bile supplements.*

Whatever the reason, your body is no longer doing what it is supposed to with your bile. The best way to fix this rapidly is with supplementation. For starters I recommend getting 2 bottles of plain old Ox Bile (yum!). Go do it, now. You can order it on online. You may not use them right away but you will want to have them on hand when you are ready to begin your digestive experiments after reading this book.

There are many over-the-counter bile supplements made either from identical chemicals (bile salts or bile acids) or real bile extracted from animals. A current list of suppliers and manufacturers (as of 2011) can be found in the index.

Figuring out the right dosage of these supplements is key to returning your system to normal. It will take several weeks of experimentation to find the right dosage and balance, as everyone is different. You may find they do not help you at all. That's ok; there are other things you can do.

There are pluses and minuses to bile supplementation. The first negative: your stomach needs to be an acid-rich environment in order to properly dissolve the food you eat. It can't do its job without the right mix.

Bile acts as an acid reducer. Putting bile into the

stomach will tend to counteract the acid-- it would be like taking your gall bladder out and putting it in front of your stomach. As a result, your stomach may need to overproduce acid, and this acid-rich mix has the potential to irritate your bowels, your stomach, and/or cause acid reflux. Too much acid in the system can cause overpopulation of bacteria in your bowels and add to the gas problem. Some manufacturers of bile supplements include some acid in the tablets to try and make up for this problem.

To the best of my knowledge, nobody makes an enteric-coated tablet designed to last just long enough to pass through the stomach intact and then dissolve in the small intestine. Which would be perfect for people like us. Is anyone listening?

The second negative: Bile also acts as a laxative and dehydrator. Too much bile in the system will definitely help "move things along" by pulling water from your intestines where it supposed to be absorbed. You don't want that.

The positive: You cannot overdose on bile, and once you get the dosage right, you will know how to reduce the urgency, liquidity, or gassiness issues you used to suffer from. You can then truly return to your previous happy existence.


### *Step 5: Supplement your diet with short- and medium-chain fatty acids.*

These fats do not require processing in your digestive tract and can be absorbed directly. You can get these in supplement form, or also by increasing your intake of the following sources:

- ☐ Butter
- ☐ Coconut Oil
- ☐ Palm Kernel Oil
- ☐ Milk fat from cow, goat, sheep, or horse
- ☐ Supplements in pill form, available at nutrition stores.

### Step 6: Take a few blood tests to check for liver and pancreatic dysfunction.

A simple range of blood tests can tell you a lot about what is going on chemically inside your body. If your liver is not in proper shape, its lack of bile production or improper chemical mixing of bile may be to blame for your gallstones.

Your pancreas could also be partly to blame. Bile must flow out through a common duct with the pancreas, and if the pancreas has problems, it may cause issues up the line with the biliary system.

All of these parts of you work together in concert, driven by hormonal signals in the bloodstream. Not only are they driven by hormones, they also produce hormones. If they are not in proper tune, the whole system gets thrown off.

These blood tests will give you a good detailed peek into the world of the liver and pancreas, and help you diagnose where your digestive imbalances need to be corrected.

*The list of blood tests is as follows:*

☐ Basic Metabolic Panel (overall health)

☐ Complete Blood Count (overall health and liver)

☐ Amylase Screen (checks pancreatic function)

☐ Hepatic Function Panel (checks liver function)

☐ Prothrombin Time (checks for liver damage and vitamin deficiency)

For specifics on these blood tests, what they contain, and what it means, see chapter 7, "What's in your blood?"

## Step 7: Consider and investigate possible food allergies.

It is entirely possible that food allergies can be to blame for (1) formation of gallstones and loss of gall bladder, and (2) post-surgery issues with indigestion, malabsorption, vitamin deficiencies, and diarrhea.

At its core, an allergy is an overblown immune response to something you came in contact with. Coeliac Disease qualifies as just one of these allergies. We know about Coeliac Disease and call it by this name simply because wheat is such a large part of modern life, but there are thousands of ingredients other than wheat out there, causing similar consequences and wreaking digestive havoc upon the innocent.

You could have a food allergy for your entire life and never know it. A food allergy need not make you immediately or extremely ill, and in fact, in a sick twist of fate, the human body has a tendency to crave foods it is allergic to.

A food allergy isn't confined to a specific food: pizza, for example. It is a reaction to a specific chemical within the food, typically individual proteins. The most common food allergies are peanuts, milk, eggs, tree nuts (walnuts, almonds, etc), fish, shellfish, soy, and wheat. The truth is that you could have or could develop a food allergy to anything.

The biological results of food allergies can be very similar to Coeliac Disease. Moreover, just like Coeliac Disease, if you do turn out to have a food allergy and stop eating what ails you, your system should slowly heal and return to its former glory. For more in-depth information on food allergies, see page 69, "Food Allergies."

### Step 8: If applicable, learn how to diagnose and prevent future gallstones.

If you still have a gall bladder, you can reduce your risk of future gallstone formation and attacks. Familiarize yourself with the risk multipliers, and the diagnostic methods and treatments discussed later.

### Step 9: Spread the knowledge.

You're not the only one with gall bladder problems. You don't have to be the only one who triumphed over them either. Granted, it's not considered polite to openly discuss our poop issues at dinner or at parties (unless it's with medical people and then all bets are off on who can gross out the others) but when you do run into other people with missing gall bladders, pass on what you have learned.

### *So now what can I expect?*

Post-surgery, you will probably notice...

☐ Weight loss. Since you are no longer as efficient in absorbing calorie-dense fats, even though you may be ingesting plenty of calories, you are not processing them well enough. These excess fats and unabsorbed calories come out in your stool, in the form of...

☐ Diarrhea and soft stool, sometimes urgent: If your stools float in the toilet, odds are that they are doing so because they are rich in fat. Normal healthy stools should be fairly firm and sink or be neutrally buoyant. Stools that float, break apart in the water and leave "graffiti" in the bowl as they flush are surefire indications that your digestive balance has been compromised. We don't want too many floaters. You may also experience...

☐ Abdominal pain and bloating. This is caused by any number of reasons from indigestion to bacterial overgrowth to bowel spasms. It will likely be accompanied by...

☐ Tremendously horrible gas the likes of which you have never before experienced. Not just volume but potency. Curl-your-nose-hairs kind of stuff that makes your spouse claw at the doors to get outside for fresh air. You will also learn that the gas is often accompanied by one or many of the other symptoms described. Never trust a fart, ever again.

21

☐ Anal leakage can also be a problem. It's caused by that constant bile outflow. This will, hopefully, eventually pass. It takes time. Hence the step 1 recommendation.

☐ Cravings for fatty foods: This is natural, as your body can no longer process them easily, it wants more volume passed through it to make up for the malabsorption. Despite the fact that you consciously know the fatty foods are going to cause you digestive upset, your body chemistry is screaming for more fats.

☐ Thirst: You may find yourself to be unusually thirsty, as in constantly toting a thermos, water bottle, etc. Especially if you suffer from PCS or Habba Syndrome (discussed in later chapters). This is because of the water you lose in diarrhea.

Well, that's certainly depressing!!! But what you may find good to know is that most of these symptoms can be prevented once you know what is happening and why, and you can take the appropriate countermeasures. This is covered in detail in the various chapters that follow.

### What to expect Physiologically:

When the gall bladder is no longer around, under normal circumstances, bile will tend to back up a bit in the bile ducts, held in by the Sphincter of Oddi. Due to this pressure, over time, there will be an enlargement of the bile ducts as a result. This is not a bad thing, and will end up working to store more bile, almost like a mini-gall-bladder. The amount of time it takes to enlarge varies from person to person. It will never hold as much as the gall bladder once did, however.

Also, once the bile ducts have held back as much as they can, the only choice your system has to deal with the extra is to let it flow out into your intestine. This can cause irritation, pH imbalances, changes in the population of intestinal bacteria, and general mayhem in your guts. If you have a bile malabsorption problem (ie the bile is not being readily absorbed in the Ileum for whatever reason) then you may experience Dumping Syndrome, Habba Syndrome, PCS, uncontrollable diarrhea, or anal leakage. I've been there. Black underpants help.

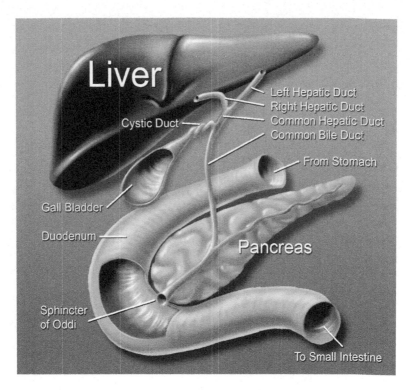

# 4: The Gall Bladder and You

The gall bladder is a small pear-shaped organ located beneath the liver. Adult gall bladders are normally 8cm long and 4cm wide when full, about the size of a deflated party balloon. A typical adult gall bladder is made to store 50 mL of concentrated bile (1.7 fl oz or about 3.5 tablespoons).

It is attached physically to the junction of the common hepatic duct (from which the liver produces bile) and the common bile duct (through which bile flows to the duodenum, or highest portion of the small intestine, alongside the pancreatic duct). Between this junction and the body of the bladder itself is a twisted passage of spiral valves called the cystic duct.

This whole arrangement of plumbing is called the "biliary tree" as it resembles a series of branches. Gall stones can form in and become trapped in any part of the bladder or biliary tree; however they are most commonly formed inside the bladder itself as that is where bile is concentrated, increasing the chances that it will crystallize.

The liver only produces bile in a slow, steady trickle. However, when you eat, bile needs to be released in a large amount in a short time span. Thus, the job of the gall bladder is to gather, store, and concentrate the bile so that it can be released quickly. As it holds the bile, it removes water from the solution, taking in 400-800ml of raw bile daily and increasing its potency, typically, by a factor of five. This heavy concentration makes it more effective in emulsifying fats in your food when it is released into the intestine after eating (for more detail on bile and what it does, see the following chapter).

The gall bladder receives its signal to release bile from the hormone Cholecystokynin, or CCK. CCK is released by the duodenum in reaction to the presence of fats passed on from the contents of your food. This CCK reaction is reduced or nullified in those suffering from Coeliac Disease, and can cause gall bladder "laziness" or complete failure to squeeze out its contents.

Unfortunately, most of the time someone begins having problems with gallstones, the preferred treatment of the day is to "cut and run" by simply removing the organ causing the problems. The medical/insurance system in the US does not exactly encourage giving doctors adequate time to properly assess, experiment on, and treat the myriad things that can cause gallstones.

Furthermore, by the time we find out what is actually going on, it is often too late, the gall bladder has become badly infected or scarred beyond repair, and must be removed.

# 5: Grade School Digestive Review

To understand the Gall Bladder's small but important role in the digestive process, it is necessary to have a basic overview of the whole system. Most of it is elementary stuff you forgot in grade school, so let's do a quick and painless review:

You eat your food, surprise surprise, and when you swallow it, it slides down the...

1. Esophagus, where it makes its way further down into the...

2. Stomach, where acids and churning action break it down into a more liquid consistency and then it is passed into the...

3. Duodenum, where bile and is added to the mix in order to (a) reduce the acid level of the contents of the stomach, and (b) emulsify fats so they can begin to be broken down. Pancreatic enzymes are also released here to aid in the breakdown of food. Then everything moves along to the...

4. Jejunum, the longest part of the small intestine, where most sugars, amino acids, and peptides are absorbed. The rest moves on to the...

5. Ileum, where the final breakdown of proteins and carbohydrates takes place, fat soluble vitamins are absorbed, and the bile injected into the Duodenum is re-absorbed and shipped back to the liver. The leftovers move on to the...

6. Large Intestine, whose main job is to extract water from the mix and then hold the waste until you are ready to expel it.

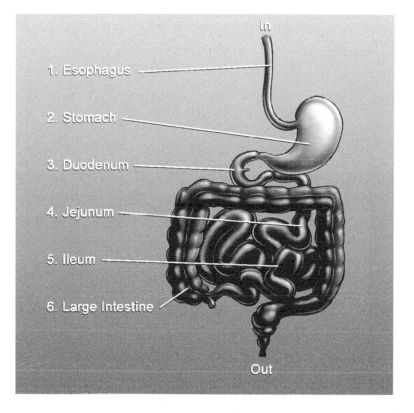

# 6: Gallstones

The specific causes of gallstone formation are still, believe it or not, somewhat of a mystery. Any of the contributing factors of individual body chemistry, weight, diet, gallbladder activity/movement, and genetics can play a part in the formation of gall stones. In other words, NOBODY KNOWS. There are too many variables. Not exactly comforting.

What can be said for certain is that at some point, the bile is not retaining all of its components in concentration (it is chemically off-balance). As the gall bladder removes water from the bile and concentrates it, certain elements in the off-balance solution begin to crystallize into grains and sediment, which build up and eventually form a stone.

It does not help much that the gall bladder is poorly engineered, resembling a deflated balloon held up by its opening. Things that solidify inside it will tend to gravitate to the bottom and stay there.

Gallstones are most commonly made up of two types of material: cholesterol and pigments. While they are always a mix of both, what classifies a stone as one or the other has to do with what material makes up the majority of the stone.

Cholesterol-based stones are more frequent than pigment stones. People with a high blood-cholesterol content are at higher risk, as the liver pulls this out of the system to make bile. Higher concentrations of cholesterol in the blood ends up as higher concentrations of cholesterol in the bile, which ends up forming into gallstones.

Pigment-based stones come from bilirubin and calcium salts which are waste byproducts of other processes in the body, filtered out by the liver and pushed down the hepatic ducts with the other bile components. People with sickle-cell anemia are more likely to have these type of stones.

## Gallstone attacks (*aka biliary colic*):

When you eat food containing fat, your gall bladder receives a hormonal battle cry from the small intestine, asking it to squeeze its contents out into the bile duct (and therefore into the small intestine). During this process a stone may be drawn up in the flow and get stuck anywhere in the biliary tree, usually at the entrance/exit of the bladder itself. This causes not only back-pressure within the gall bladder due to the bile's inability to exit the bladder, but in addition the bladder's lining rubbing against the stone can cause inflammation, scarring, and eventually infection. After a while, the gall bladder relaxes and the stone settles back away from the opening. It may not get stuck again for some time.

Smaller stones which manage to leave the bladder may become lodged in other parts of the biliary tree. If the pancreatic duct becomes blocked, the lucky recipient of the gallstone may also develop pancreatitis, described as possibly the worst pain one can experience. Fun!

After enough repeated gallstone attacks, the gall bladder will be so beat up, scarred, and infected that it fails to work properly at all. At this point it will have to be removed. This is what happened to mine.

## Statistics:

☐ Women are twice as likely as men to form gallstones.

☐ There is a politically incorrect indicator for gallstone risk called "The Four F's: Fat, Female, Fertile, Forty". In other words, women over forty years of age who have had multiple children and are overweight are in the highest risk category.

☐ Gallstones are colorblind and treat all races with equal contempt. However for unknown reasons, Scandinavians are more susceptible than average, as are the Pima tribe of Native Americans who have a genetic predisposition. Interestingly, the Pimas of Mexico do not suffer to the extent that their northern counterparts do, mainly due to diet.

☐ People with direct relatives who had gallstones are more than four times more at risk than the average person. (my grandmother had her gall bladder removed and my mother has asymptomatic gallstones; great grandpa Stanley died in 1941 from complications after his gall bladder surgery)

☐ People with Coeliac Disease (also spelled Celiac Disease) are almost guaranteed to suffer from gall bladder dysfunction and are also at higher risk of forming gallstones as a result.

☐ Obese/overweight people usually have a higher risk of stones due to the often correlating higher levels of blood cholesterol.

☐ Diabetics and people with Metabolic Syndrome or

Sickle Cell Anemia have a higher risk of gallstones.

☐ People who have recently undergone rapid weight loss have higher risk of gallstones.

# Identifying Gallstones

Though most gallstones cannot easily be seen on x-rays, there are a variety of other ways to find them.

## *ERCP:*

An ERCP, or cholangiogram (or its long name Endoscopic Retrograde Cholangio-Pancreatography) can be done by inserting an endoscope down your throat and into your intestine, using it to inject radio-opaque dye up into the bile duct and then taking x-rays of the abdomen. The advantage to this procedure is that the endoscope can be used to remove small stones, or place a stent (reinforcing tube) in a clogged duct to keep it open. This is the same procedure described in the "gall bladder treatments" section later on, only here it is being used to assess the situation for treatment. It is entirely possible that the assessment and treatment can be done during the same procedure using the same scope.

## *HIDA scan:*

A gall bladder radionuclide scan (also known as cholescintigraphy or a HIDA scan) works in a similar fashion but with an intravenous needle. Radioactive dye is injected into a vein, makes its way to the liver, and is ultimately flushed into the bile ducts, making the stones visible in a gamma-sensitive camera.

### MRI/MRCP:

An MRI scan, or more specifically an MRCP (Magnetic Resonance Cholangio-Pancreatography) uses an MRI machine to scan your bile system to find stones. It requires no injections and is just as accurate as the other scans. You lay on a table which slides you into the machine, you get scanned, and out you go. No drugs, no needles, no scopes down your throat.

### Ultrasound:

An ultrasound can easily spot gallstones, requires no drugs or needles, can be done in a matter of minutes, and can be done affordably at any ultrasound clinic in the world; no need to go to a big hospital.

The MRI/MRCP and ultrasound methods also have the advantages of being able to check the thickness of the gall bladder's walls and therefore gauge the level of inflammation or infection it may have.

# Gallstone Symptoms

The first symptom of gallstones is "biliary colic" which is the pain caused by gallstones blocking the bile duct. The pain is not localized; in other words you cannot really pinpoint where it is coming from, other than in your abdomen. It just plain hurts. It is triggered most often with the eating of fatty foods; because the gall bladder goes into overdrive to deal with the fats, the stones tend to get shoved into the small exit at the cystic duct and jam up the exit. The bladder then continues to squeeze, grinding the stone into the cystic duct as it tries in vain to get its bile out, causing you vast amounts of pain and discomfort.

The next stage is cholecystis, or inflammation of the gall bladder. This is caused by irritation from the presence of the gallstones and their duct-blocking tendencies.

The inflammation and the presence of gallstones then cause thickening of the bile (inspissation) which is a recipe for growing and/or more numerous gallstones, and bile stasis (bile which cannot escape or cycle properly) which leads to secondary infection by the bacteria living in the digestive tract. When the gall bladder is not working properly, which at this point it is not, it is called *biliary dyskinesia*. This is the state that precedes gangrene. Gangrene is, literally, *rot,* from the inside out, and it *will kill you.*

It's really not nice in there at this point, so if you do catch gallstones early, before your gall bladder is compromised, do have them treated as quickly as you can.

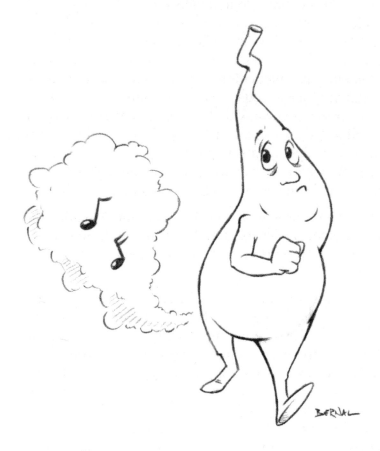

# 7: Gallstone treatments

If you are fortunate enough to have caught your gallstone problem before your gall bladder was ruined, you have a few options for treatment.

## *ERCP:*

If this sounds familiar from the diagnostic list that's because it is the same procedure involving the same equipment, only this refers to using it to treat the stones after they are found. ERCP or "Endoscopic Retrograde Cholangio-Pancreatoscopy" (say that 5 times fast!) can be used not only to assess the situation in your gall bladder but can be used to treat the problem as well. Using this procedure, some stones can be removed from the gall bladder or bile duct without the need for surgery. Basically the doctor runs a fancy endoscope down your throat and then up through the ducts from which your bile flows, and dissolves the stones with chemicals injected by the scope. With this procedure, you do not need to be opened up with knives, and the doctor will have a camera's-eye view of the inside of your bile ducts and gall bladder, by which he/she can further assess just how bad the situation may be.

### Bile Acid Supplementation:

Some stones can be treated with oral ingestion of bile acid. This has a roughly 75% rate of success on cholesterol-based stones, but 15% of the patients of this treatment still end up with recurring gallstones within 2-3 years.

### Lithotripsy:

The use of sonic shock waves, or Lithotripsy, to break up gallstones can be very effective . This treatment is good in that it does not require the patient to be anesthetized, however repeated treatments will be necessary to ensure that the stones have all been broken down into small enough pieces that they can be passed through the bile duct without getting stuck. Patients with a single stone have much higher success rates than patients with multiple stones. 95% of stones treated this way are passed within 12-18 months. This treatment does increase the risk of pancreatitis and gall bladder inflammation (acute cholecystitis) because the small pieces still need to pass through the bile ducts and can cause irritation along the way.

## Contact Dissolution:

Another more meat-and-potatoes way to get rid of gallstones is "contact dissolution" which involves injecting chemicals directly into the gall bladder by way of a percutaneous catheter (a really long needle) to dissolve the stones. In cases with multiple gallstones, this method is the most effective, with a 95% success rate. MTBE (methyl tertiary-butyl ether) is commonly used as the solvent. Side effects are caused by the body's absorption of the MTBE and can include vomiting, difficulty breathing, drowsiness, and bad breath. Of course you also have to deal with having a needle stuck into you for 5-12 hours for the treatment so anesthesia, while preferable, is not mandatory. But you get to keep your gall bladder.

## Cholecystectomy:

And, last but not least, a 100% effective way to remove gall stones is to cut you open and take the whole gall bladder out. This involves sedating the patient and using a laparoscope to dig out the pesky organ. In most cases the patient can go home the same day of the procedure and resume normal life within a few days.

In the old days, removing a gall bladder was a critical and barbaric procedure which had an uncomfortable probability of killing the patient from the procedure, not to mention the complications of the long recovery. This is what killed Great Grandpa Stanley. Be glad for modern medical tools!

# 8: What's in your Blood?

Blood tests can go a long way in diagnosing problems with minimal cost. They are an easy way to see what's going on inside your body via analysis of chemicals and other indicators of health. All of these blood tests will require at least 12 hours of fasting before drawing the blood sample.

☐ A **CBC (Complete Blood Count)** screen checks for any disease or infections. Anything outside the normal ranges may be cause for concern. High RBC counts tend to indicate kidney and liver diseases. Low RBC counts tend to indicate stomach ulcers and IBS (Inflammatory Bowel Disease). Normal ranges are as follows:

☐ White Blood Cell (WBC):
*Men and nonpregnant women:*
4,500–11,000/mcL$^3$ or 4.5–11.0 x $10^9$/L
*Pregnant women:*
1st trimester: 6,600–14,100/mcL or 6.6–14.1 x $10^9$/L
2nd trimester: 6,900–17,100/mcL or 6.9–17.1 x $10^9$/L
3rd trimester: 5,900–14,700/mcL or 5.9–14.7 x $10^9$/L
Postpartum: 9,700–25,700/mcL or 9.7–25.7 x $10^9$/L

☐ Red Blood Cell (RBC):
*Men:*
4.7–6.1 million RBCs/mcL or 4.7–6.1 x $10^{12}$/L
*Women:*
4.2–5.4 million RBCs/mcL or 4.2–5.4 x $10^{12}$/L

43

- Hematocrit (HCT):
  *Men:*
  42%–52% or 0.42–0.52 volume fraction
  *Women:*
  37%–47% or 0.37–0.47 volume fraction
  *Pregnant women:*
  1st trimester: 35%–46%
  2nd trimester: 30%–42%
  3rd trimester: 34%–44%
  Postpartum: 30%–44%

- Hemoglobin (Hgb):
  *Men:*
  14–18 g/dL or 8.7–11.2 mmol/L
  *Women:*
  12–16 g/dL or 7.4–9.9 mmol/L
  *Pregnant Women:*
  1st trimester: 11.4–15.0 g/dL or 7.1–9.3 mmol/L
  2nd trimester: 10.0–14.3 g/dL or 6.2–8.9 mmol/L
  3rd trimester: 10.2–14.4 g/dL or 6.3–8.9 mmol/L
  Postpartum: 10.4–18.0 g/dL or 6.4–9.3 mmol/L

- Red Blood Cell Indices:
  Mean Corpuscular Volume (MVC): 82-89 femtoliters (fL)
  Mean Corpuscular Hemoglobin (MCH): 26-34 picograms (pg)
  Mean Corpuscular Hemoglobin Concentration (MCHC): 31-38 grams per deciliter (g/dL) or 31-38%

- Red Cell Distribution Width (RDW):
  11.5-14.6%

- Platelet (Thrombocyte) Count:
  150,000–400,000 platelets per $mm^3$ or 150–400 x $10^9$/L

- Mean Platelet Volume (MPV):
  7.4–10.4 $mcm^3$ or 7.4–10.4 fL

☐ **Basic Metabolic Panel (BMP)** This typically includes blood chemical tests for:

☐ Sodium (NA+)
Normal range: 137.- 147 mmol/L

☐ Potassium (K+)
Normal range: 3.4 - 5.3 mmol/L

☐ Chloride (Cl-)
Normal range: 99 - 108 mmol/L

☐ Bicarbonate (HCO3-) or CO2
Normal range: 22 - 29 mmol/L

☐ Blood Urea Nitrogen (BUN)
Normal range: 8 - 21 mg/dL

☐ Creatinine
Normal range male: 0.6 - 1.3 mg/dL
Normal range female: 0.5 - 1.1 mg/dL

☐ Glocose
Normal range fasting: 60 - 109 mg/dL
Normal range nonfasting: 60 - 200 mg/dL

☐ Calcium (Ca2+)
Normal: 8.7 - 10.7 mg/dL

☐ **Amylase screen** to check for pancreatic disease.
Blood test normal range: 23 to 85 u/L (units/Liter)
Urine test normal range: 2.6 to 21.2 IU/h (int'l units per hour)

☐ **Hepatic Function Panel (HFP)** to check the status of your liver function. Normal ranges are as follows:

☐ Total Protein: 6.0 – 8.4 gm/dL.
Elevated levels may indicate dehydration and high levels of albumin and/or globulin. Low total protein levels can indicate a liver or kidney disorder.

☐ Albumin: 3.5 – 5.0 gm/dL.
Elevated levels of albumin may indicate dehydration. Low levels of albumin may indicate liver disease, nephrotic syndrome, heart failure or low intake or absorption of protein.

☐ Total Bilirubin: up to 1.0 mg/dL.
Elevated levels may indicate hepatitis, cirrhosis, neoplasm, alcoholism, hemolytic disease, biliary obstruction or anorexia. Low levels are nothing to worry about.

☐ Direct Bilirubin: up to 0.4 mg/dL.
Elevated levels may indicate hepatitis, cirrhosis, neoplasm or biliary disease. Low levels are nothing to worry about.

☐ Alkaline Phosphatase: 50 – 160 units/L.
Elevated levels may indicate bone growth or disease, liver disease, malignancies in the bone and liver or leukemia. Low levels may indicate a zinc deficiency, hypothyroidism, Vitamin C deficiency, excessive Vitamin D intake, malnutrition or Vitamin B6 deficiency.

☐ AST: 7 – 27 units/L.
Elevated levels may indicate alcoholism, cirrhosis, hepatitis, drug therapy or biliary disease. Low levels may indicate uremia, Vitamin B6 deficiency or drug therapy.

☐ ALT: 1 – 21 units/L.
Elevated levels may indicate liver disease, hepatocyte injury, hepatitis, drug therapy or biliary disease. Low levels are nothing to worry about.

☐ **Prothrombin Time (PT)** which is a test of blood's clotting abilities (coagulation), an indicator of Vitamin K status and a way to check for possible liver damage. Normal range for prothrombin time is 12–15 seconds, and the normal range for INR (International normalized ratio) is 0.8–1.2.

☐ **Antibody testing for Coeliac Disease:**

☐ IgA/tTG antibody check:

Sensitivity 90%, Specificity 99%. IgA means anti-transglutamase antibodies. IgA is also called tTG (tissue trans-glutamase). If your test comes back IgA positive, there is a 97% chance that you have Coeliac Disease. This test does give occasional false-negatives; if you test negative, there is only a 71% chance that the negative result is accurate. This is why you should also do the next test at the same time...

☐ IgG anti-gliadin antibody check:

Sensitivity 87%, Specificity 91%. This test shows positive results more readily but does not have as strong a correlation to proving Coeliac Disease. For ecample, IgG-positive results show up in 21% of people suffering from non-Coeliac digestive disorders. This test may not provide as good a test-positive result

47

as the IgA/tTG but it provides less false-negatives, and therefore should be done at the same time.

# 9: The Secret World of Bile

Most never see it. Or those who have seen it probably weren't paying attention (like everyone's first truly Biblical hangover where they had to spend a day hugging the toilet, when the stomach had run out of alcohol and other food contents, and bile was all that was left to throw up). To truly understand bile, we must first learn where it comes from, and then move on to what it does.

Bile is produced by hepatocytes in the liver. A hepatocyte is a cell which synthesizes and stores protein, synthesizes cholesterol, bile salts, and phospholipids, transforms carbohydrates, and generally filters out all sorts of nasty crap that ends up in your blood stream. Hepatocytes make up 70-80% of the liver's mass.

The liver is basically your body's largest chemical sorting and manufacturing factory. Anything useful it pulls from the bloodstream, processes, and ships out in another form that the other parts of the body need. Anything it can't use, it dumps out as waste into the hepatic ducts, and that material becomes bile.

During the creation of bile, salty compounds and electrolytes are added to the flow which both dilute and increase the alkalinity of the solution (alkalines are the opposites of acids). This chemical cocktail then flows down the hepatic ducts and is stored in the gall bladder, which collects and holds it until it is called up for its release by the hormonal trigger Cholecystokinin (CCK), which comes from the duodenum when it senses the presence of fats in your food.

The human liver can produce up to 1 liter (roughly 1 quart) of bile per day, though the average is 400-800mL, about the volume of a soda can. This volume is reduced when the gall bladder concentrates it, by around a factor of 5. Any surplus bile not able to be stored in the gall bladder simply has no other choice but to flow out into the small intestine, but in most cases this does not happen unless the gall bladder has been compromised or removed.

Malabsorption of fats is the primary problem we face after we lose our gall bladders-- the chemical nutrients in fats simply cannot be broken up efficiently without the proper amount of bile, and that proper amount of bile is absent if the gall bladder cannot dump it out in quantity when you eat. This excess fat in the digestive tract can cause irritation, urgent bowel movements, gassiness, diarrhea, and soft stool. Excess bile in the digestive tract can also cause similar problems. Finding a balance is critical, and difficult, especially if your gall bladder is missing-in-action.

Another unfortunate side-effect with inadequate bile volume is that fat-soluble vitamins such as A, D, E, and K are not as readily absorbed, and this can cause deficiencies. These vitamins can *only* be absorbed in the presence of fat, which can *only* be moved through the cell wall of the intestine efficiently with the breakdown action of bile salts.

The alkalinity of the bile salts aids in neutralizing stomach acid in the small intestine. Bile salts are also bactericidal, and are responsible for killing off many of the bugs that enter the digestive tract in your food. If your bile output is reduced, the higher acidity of your intestinal contents and lowered bactericidal properties of the bile will throw off the population balance of the types of healthy and unhealthy bacteria that live in your digestive system, leading to gassiness and loss of important nutrients to hungry bacteria.

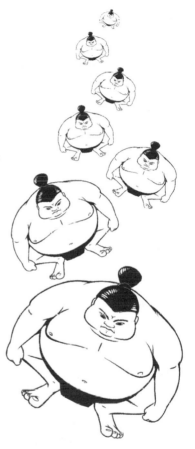

Just like any other nutrient, your body needs fats. And just like any other nutrient, too much or too little can cause problems. Now that your gall bladder is not doing its job, you need to pay careful attention to not only your fat intake, but how those fats are being dealt with in your digestive system.

To better understand the whole process, let's take a bizarre trip down into the feudal lands of your intestines, and meet the cast of characters that lives there and how they interact with the introduction of fats in your food.

The story could not begin, of course, without fat. Fats are necessary. The body needs them to repair itself, to produce hormones, to burn for energy and to store for future energy. The liver can synthesize fats from other dietary components but it must take those components from somewhere-- first it taps the supply of nutrients in your bloodstream, and then it starts to pull from other parts of the body (muscle, bone, etc). So in order to keep from consuming yourself, you must ingest and *absorb* fats and fatty acids. For us, ingesting them is never a problem. It is absorbing them that is difficult.

Your body cannot absorb fats in their natural form. If it could, we wouldn't need bile, we wouldn't need a gall bladder, you wouldn't be reading this, I wouldn't be writing this, and we'd both be swimming in greasy double-cheeseburgers with bacon and chili-cheese fries.

Fats cannot be absorbed directly through the wall of the intestine; the molecules are too big and not the right type. They need to be broken down into smaller pieces first. We therefore need a tool to break the fats down into things that *can* be absorbed into the intestinal wall.

The tool we use to break down fats is Lipase, an enzyme produced by the pancreas and released into the duodenum (small intestine) through the Sphincter of Oddi, the same passage through which bile flows from its ducts and gall bladder.

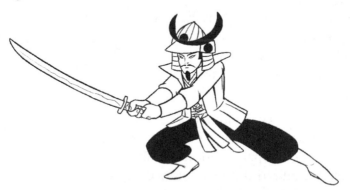

Meet the Lipase Samurai.

The Lipase Samurai is one of many Enzymes whose job it is to cut complex molecules into smaller parts that can be easily absorbed by your body. Lipase Samurai has just one job: he attacks Fat Sumo globules and chops them into smaller water-soluble components.

If the Lipase Samurai did not exist, the army of Fat Sumos would stomp right on through your intestine, causing terrible diarrhea. In addition you would miss out on the valuable nutrients they contain.

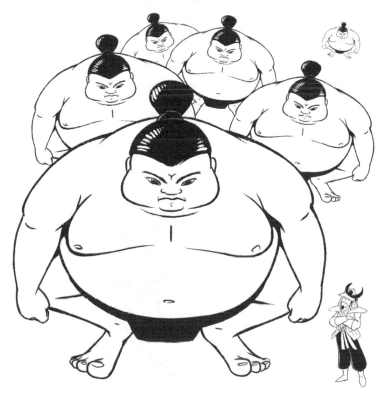

The Lipase Samurai's job is not easy, because fat molecules are sticky and have a tendency to group together to form large fat droplets like our Giant Fat

Sumo. These large fat droplets have a low surface area compared to their high volume, so it is extremely difficult for the Lipase Samurai to chop them into their component parts. If the Giant Fat Sumo was smaller, the Lipase Samurai could actually deal him some damage.

Fortunately he has a whole army of Bile Salt Ninjas, whose job it is to pull Giant Fat Sumos apart into smaller pieces. These Ninjas are stored in your gall bladder until they hear the battle cry of the Cholecystokinin (CCK) hormone, which is released by the Duodenum (the first segment of the small intestine) when it detects the presence of Fat Sumos.

Bile Salts are interesting molecules in that one side repels water (hydrophobic) and one side attracts water (hydrophilic). The neat thing about the hydrophobic side of the Bile Salt is that not only does it repel water, but it acts like a magnet to fat. This attribute makes them excellent at emulsifying (separating and dispersing), big sticky Giant Sumo Fat particles into smaller pieces which the Lipase Samurai can fight.

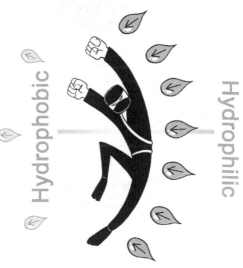

54

Once a group of our Bile Salt Ninjas comes into contact with a Giant Fat Sumo (1), they will tend to surround him with their hydrophobic side and and push/pull him apart into smaller and smaller droplets with their hydrophilic side (2). This increases the surface area while reducing the volume of each Fat Sumo globule.

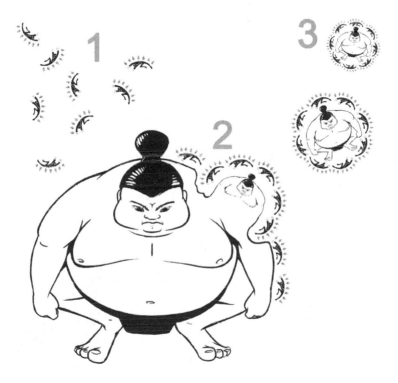

The end result is that big Giant Fat Sumo globules are broken into several Small Fat Sumo globules surrounded by a layer of Bile Salt Ninjas, which are then surrounded by a jacket of water. This molecular formation is known as a Micelle (3).

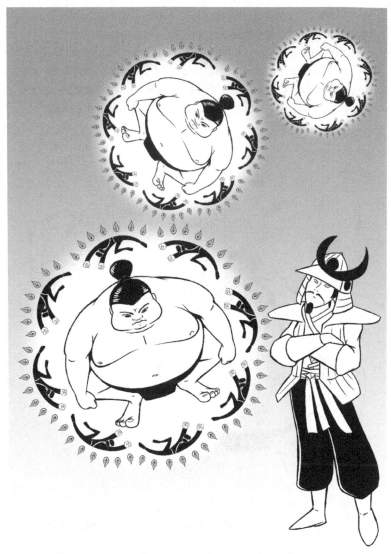

Now the Fat Sumo has been reduced to many
smaller size pieces that the Lipase Samurai can handle.

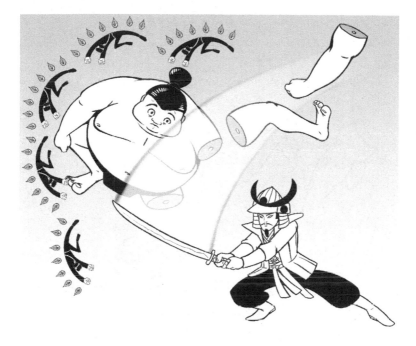

The Lipase Samurai jumps in between his Bile Salt Ninja friends and slices the Fat Sumo into Fatty Acids and Monoglycerides.

Fatty Acids are an important source of energy because they contain relatively large quantities of ATP, the basic fuel of cellular life.

Any animal fats you ingest will contain various amounts of cholesterol, which your body needs to form and maintain cell walls, process and synthesize vitamins, and to build steroids and sex hormones. Ingesting animal fats is very important.

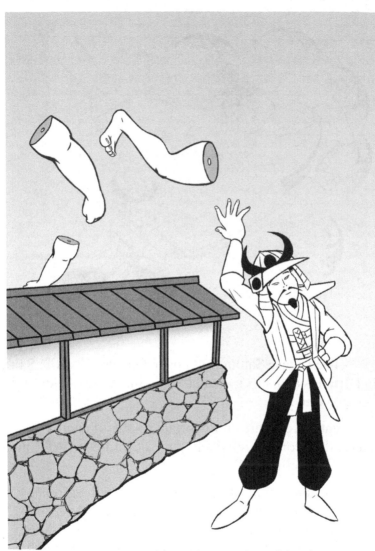

These Fatty Acid and Monoglyceride pieces can now be passed through the cell wall of the intestine and into the bloodstream, where they are shipped off to parts of the body that need them, or sent to the liver to be processed into other things.

Once the bile salts have done their job, they are re-absorbed by the intestinal wall of the Ileum (the third and final portion of the small intestine) and sent back via the bloodstream to your liver, to be re-secreted as more bile. Sometimes the same bile molecules will make the cycle up to 3 times in a single meal.

We need fats and we need fat-soluble vitamins for our bodies to work properly. When the gall bladder is no longer doing its job, either because it is blocked or because it is not there at all anymore, the body is no longer getting proper nutrition, the whole system is set off-balance, and lots of bad things can result.

Your body still produces bile, fortunately. Unfortunately, something is wrong with its release: Without a gall bladder, it is not only being leaked constantly into your intestines when it shouldn't be, but it is no longer in ample supply when you need it (ie: during a meal). With a dysfunctional gall bladder, similar results occur but only because the bladder itself is already full and refuses to cooperate because it's not being told to get to work.

Once your biliary system is off-balance, it is now performing an inadequate job at its primary task of coming out in force to emulsify the fats in your meal, and is also actively sabotaging the rest of your digestive process by drawing too much water into the digestive tract when it has no fats to attack.

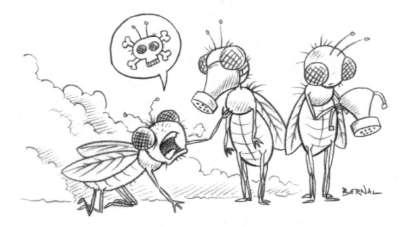

60

# 10: Symptoms, Syndromes, and other Mayhem

When your digestive system's balance is thrown off, either by an uncooperative or missing organ, you can and may experience all manner of unpleasant side effects. Those described here are by no means a complete list but are representative of the most common.

### *Biliary Reflux:*
aka Bile Reflux, or Duodenogastric Reflux. This occurs when bile flows backwards/upwards in the digestive tract from the duodenum into the stomach and/or esophagus. If this is chronic it should definitely not go untreated, as the bile will reduce the effectiveness of stomach acid and make an excellent environment for bacterial infections and ulcers. Symptoms include frequent heartburn, nausea, and vomiting bile. Causes include damage to the pyloric sphincter from surgery, peptic ulcers, or gall bladder surgery.

### *Habba Syndrome:*
This is a syndrome that affects both pre- and post-surgical patients. The most noticeable symptom of this syndrome is urgent and often uncontrollable diarrhea following meals. See the post-surgery chapter for more detailed information on Habba Syndrome.

### Vitamin Deficiency:

Vitamins A, D, E, and K need to hitchhike through the intestinal wall on the backs of fat molecules in order for your body to absorb them. If the fats in your digestive tract are not being properly broken down and absorbed, niether are A, D, E, or K. Your body needs these vitamins in order to function properly, and deficiencies can result in bone deterioration, drops in hormone levels, and other harmful side-effects. See the chapter "The Ugly Consequences of Malabsorption" for further details.


### Gas and Bloating:

When the balanced environment in your digestive tract changes from pH (acid concentration levels), flow, or the lack or overabundance of bile, your bacterial friends will be off balance too. They will have feast or famine, find new homes where they don't belong, new gangs will move in where the old ones moved out, and your guts will turn into a giant gas factory. Not only that, but some nutrients you require from their help in breaking down food will be passed through your system more rapidly, meaning you are not absorbing as efficiently as you once did. If their populations grow out of hand, they can even rob you of your hard-earned nutrients!


### Diarrhea:

Often accompanying gas and bloating. This needs no explanation, really. Nobody likes it but when we have a lousy or missing gall bladder we are often the unlucky recipients of diarrhea. Long term effects from chronic diarrhea are nutritional deficiencies and dehydration.

# The Coeliac Connection

Coeliac Disease (spelled Celiac in the USA) is an autoimmune disorder caused by a reaction to gliadin, a gluten protein found in wheat. The reaction causes inflammation of the small intestine, which leads to atrophy of the vilii (surface cells), which then causes malabsorption of nutrients. Coeliac Disease is not a symptom of gall bladder dysfunction, but it can definitely be a cause. If you are suffering from gall bladder problems you should definitely be screened for Coeliac Disease. It affects about 1% of the population in the USA.

Coeliac Disease gets in the way of proper gall bladder function by dampening or canceling out the CCK signal sent from the duodenum. If the duodenum can't sense fat content because its lining is inflamed or atrophied, it doesn't know to send the CCK and call the gall bladder to action.

The gall bladder, not getting the proper signal, either sits idle waiting or does an inadequate job and doesn't give 100% effort. Therefore bile doesn't circulate properly, it has a greater opportunity to settle and crystallize, and the chance of gallstone formation is greatly increased.

Not only does Coeliac Disease cause malabsorption of nutrients in general due to its inflammatory nature, but its problems are further compounded by a double dose of malabsorption caused by reduced bile output from a lazy or unresponsive gall bladder. As the atrophy of the intestinal lining worsens over time, more symptoms and digestive disorders can result (such as lactose intolerance).

**Symptoms of Coeliac Disease:**

- Diarrhea: often pale and foul-smelling
- Abdominal pain and cramping
- Bloating
- Often misdiagnosed as IBS (Irritable Bowel Syndrome)
- Vitamin A, D, E, and K deficiencies
- Calcium malabsorption/deficiency
- Bacterial overgrowth in the bowels
- Dermatitis Herpetiformis (DH), an itchy skin rash
- Mouth ulcers
- Hypothyroidism
- Iron deficiency
- Chronic fatigue
- Osteoporosis
- Intestinal cancer
- Sterility

**Getting tested for Coeliac Disease:**

Blood tests are the fastest way to screen for Coeliac Disease. The tests you should get are as follows:

☐ IgA or tTG antibodies: Sensitivity 90%, Specificity 99%. IgA means anti-transglutamase antibodies. These antibodies are very specific, occurring 100% in people with Coeliac Disease, and 80% in people with DH (Dermatitis Herpetiformis). IgA is also called tTG (tissue trans-glutamase). If your test comes back IgA positive, there is a 97% chance that you have Coeliac Disease. This test does give occasional false-negatives; if you test negative, there is only a 71% chance that the negative result is accurate.

☐ IgG anti-gliadin antibodies: Sensitivity 87%, Specificity 91%. This test shows positive results more readily but does not have as strong a correlation to proving Coeliac Disease. For ecample, IgG-positive results show up in 21% of people suffering from non-Coeliac digestive disorders. This test may not provide as good a test-positive result as the IgA/tTG but it provides less false-negatives, and therefore should be done at the same time.

Other testing methods:

☐ Endoscopy with biopsy of duodenum or jejunum. Most Coeliac sufferers have a bowel that appears normal through the endoscope but inspection of a tissue sample viewed through a microscope reveals proof of the disease.

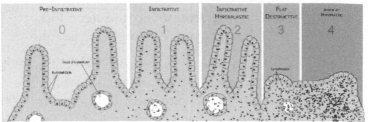

What to do if you have Coeliac Disease:

Presently, the only cure is to go on a gluten-free diet for the rest of your life. There are no miracle medications. Fortunately the solution requires only willpower, and costs nothing extra. In time, the intestinal walls will heal and the symptoms will abate or disappear completely.

Unfortunately, this means that you will have to stop ingesting anything containing gluten. The list of forbidden ingredients containing gluten is as follows:

- Wheat
- Spelt
- Kamut
- Rye
- Barley
- Triticale
- Oats (if your oats are pure, you may not need to exclude them; normally they do not contain gluten but the machines that process oats are also used to process the other grains and may be cross-

contaminated. There are also studies that show oats contain peptide sequences very similar to gluten which can cause problems in 10% of Coeliac patients)

The list does not stop there; all things derived from the above products must be avoided as well:

☐ Bread and flour products of all kinds, with exception to pure corn bread.

☐ Beer (Rest In Peace!)

☐ Most types of Whiskey

☐ Malts

*A general list of things that are gluten-free:*

☐ Corn

☐ Potatoes

☐ Rice

☐ Cassava

☐ Yams

☐ Chickpeas/garbanzo

☐ Meats (be careful of sausages, as some use ingredients containing gluten as filler or flavor enhancers)

☐ Wine, rum, brandy, sake, vodka, and other spirits derived from fruit, honey, sugar, rice, potatoes, or corn.

67

The particulars of following a gluten-free diet could easily fill their own book. There are a wealth of gluten-free diet books on the market. It is such a common problem that there is even a "Celiac Disease for Dummies" book in addition to a "Living Gluten-free for Dummies" and a "Gluten-free Cooking for Dummies." All three are quite informative, and rated 4 stars or higher on that online bookstore everyone knows.

# Food Allergies

Just like Coeliac Disease (which is itself a specific food allergy), other food allergies can cause identical problems or worse.

Most proteins are hacked to bits by the enzymatic friends of our Lipase Samurai, absorbed into the intestine, and shipped off where they need to go via the bloodstream. Some of them are not so easy to break down. Sometimes your body lacks the particular Samurai for a particular job, and certain types of proteins get past the defensive line of our Enzymatic Samurai Army. This situation is the beginning of a food allergy.

Behind the line of Enzymatic Samurai is an army of archers which shoot arrow-shaped Immunoglobin-E antibodies into these rogue proteins. The purpose of these arrows is to tag their target for later processing by the elite soldiers of your immune system.

Most of the time, your immune system keeps quiet order in the various provinces of your body, ready at any moment for a call to battle. Occasional uprisings occur but your elite immune soldiers quickly and efficiently defend you with deadly force.

When your Immune System Soldiers see a group of antibody-tagged proteins wandering around unattended, they get grumpy. The shock-and-awe campaign that they wage in retaliation for such a transgression causes collateral damage to the environment within you, sometimes so severe as to cause you serious harm, or even death.

And, once they have viewed these rogue proteins

as unwanted guests, they follow a zero-tolerance policy on anyone they encounter in the future who has similar traits.

Food allergies are categorized in 3 groups depending on the way in which antibodies play a part (or not, as may be the case).

### *Immediate hypersensitivity reaction. Can include:*

☐ Rhinitis: Itching, swelling, mucus production.

☐ Rashes and hives.

☐ Conjunctivitis (itchy red eyes)

☐ Eczema

☐ Asthma or respiratory difficulties

☐ Swelling of the throat

☐ Edema (swelling of the skin, especially around the mouth and eyes)

☐ Burning of the lips, mouth, ears, throat.

☐ Vomiting

☐ Diarrhea

☐ Severe indigestion

☐ Cramps

### *Reaction to IgE or non-IgE antibodies:*

☐ Esophagitis (swelling of the throat)

☐ Gastritis (swelling/irritation of the stomach)

☐ Gastroenteritis (swelling/irritation of the entire digestive tract)

### Caused specifically by Non-IgE antibodies:

- Food-protein-induced Entercolitis Syndrome (also called FPIES)

- Inflammation of the anus, rectum, and/or colon.

- Protein-induced enteropathy (Celiac Disease)

- Milk Soy Protein Intolerance (MSPI), mostly occurs in children.

- Heiner Syndrome (bleeding of the lungs due to a milk protein allergy)

### Other bad things that can happen from food allergies:

- Respiratory arrest

- Cardiac arrest (heart attack)

- Anaphylactic shock (both of the above, very bad)

- Serious drops in blood pressure

Odds are that if you have (or had) a serious reaction to a food allergy, you would know about it from the standard fare of immediate hypersensitivity reactions (irritation, hives, etc). The more subtle, sneaky food allergies are the ones we may have but not know about. These ones cause slow, quiet damage over a long period of time. These ones are the kind that make our gall bladders die out, and throw our digestive processes out of alignment.

Fortunately there are some simple ways to determine if you have food allergies.

### Step 1: View your cravings with extreme suspicion.

Food cravings, strangely enough, are a good indicator of things you might be allergic to. Biochemical processes in your body may be to blame, even though they end up being self-destructive.

Solving this puzzle may be as simple as looking at the things you crave. Now when I say "craving" I mean something deep in your mind that must be satisfied to the point it becomes distracting. When you just can't take it anymore and MUST have that chocolate bar... you MUST have that bacon cheeseburger... you MUST have those curly fries... you count the minutes until your break because the egg salad sandwich down at the deli is sucking away your will to live... certain things in your refrigerator have that special space because you always have it around (my Diet Coke for example), and you try to stop eating it because it's really not very good for you but you just can't quit... when all other items in your life are secondary to getting that fix of whatever it is after you wake up and have finished your morning routines, *that* is a craving.

Make mental note of the cravings you find yourself subject to, and make a physical list, on paper, of these foods. Now analyze the ingredients of these foods and see if you can find a common ingredient. It may surprise you.

Then, try giving up (just temporarily!) these addictive craving foods for a week or two and see if it makes any difference in your poop.

### Step 2: Skin prick testing.

You will have to visit an allergist for this. They will map a section of your skin (often on the arm or the back) and poke you with small needles tipped with various common allergens. These tests are by no means 100% conclusive but they should show IgE reactions and can also help confirm suspicions if you have had repeated bad experiences with specific types of food.

### Step 3: Blood testing.

Your blood can be tested in many ways to determine if you have a food allergy. The RAST (RadioAllergoSorbent Test) is a screen to check for IgE antibodies in response to specific allergens. There is a more specific type called CAP-RAST which can determine just how many antibodies are showing up for different allergens, so you know just how reactive your immune system is to various irritants. A single blood sample can be tested for several hundred allergic reactions. The downside to these tests is that it cannot be used for non-IgE antibody reactions.

### Step 4: Food challenges.

Once you have narrowed down your suspicions to a particular (or several) allergic reactions, your doctor can test you using a double-blind experiment using 2 capsules: one contains the allergen, and the other is a placebo (contains nothing). If you experience a reaction to the true allergen capsule and not the placebo, then it is pretty much proof that you are allergic to that substance.

### Step 5: Stop eating that!

This doesn't need much explanation. Once you have identified a food allergy, you will have to learn to live without this particular food for the remainder of your life. Otherwise you can cause terrible damage to your intestines.

This won't necessarily be easy. For those with wheat, egg, soy, and/or milk allergies, it may be extremely difficult just to avoid these items. Look at the ingredient list of just about any commercially available food product and it will likely contain all four. Wheat and soy are particularly difficult to avoid. During a recent trip to our deli counter, we were shocked to find that not a single deli meat behind the counter was devoid of wheat or soy. You would be amazed by just how pervasive soy is these days-- it's in EVERYTHING!

Get in the habit of checking the ingredients of everything you eat to make sure they do not contain the offending rogue proteins that cause you grief. When in doubt, go without. There are a variety of excellent online resources that can help you in making proper food decisions, such as:

[] www.Zeer.com

[] http://www.glutenfreeinfo.com

[] http://www.glutenfree.com/

Even if you do not have a wheat allergy, you may find that following a gluten-free diet, or Paleo diet, improves things. Despite the fact that I do not have Coeliac Disease, after a few weeks on a gluten-free diet, I found that my digestive situation had much improved.

I still have moments when I feel like life without bread or cookies just isn't worth living, and I break down and eat some. It's OK so long as you don't do it frequently. Just know what you are getting into, and that you will probably feel like crap after you satisfy your craving (not just morally but physically). Brownies are just too good to pass up; bring on the early grave!

# Post-Vegan Apocalypse

Randy, a former co-worker, went through a phase in his life when he ate nothing but low-fat salads and vegetables. Breakfast, lunch, and dinner. For more than a year he was steadfast and never touched meat and fatty foods.

Then, one day, he broke down and feasted on the most greasy, slimy, repulsive double cheeseburger he could find. He had an instant gallstone attack, was hospitalized, and had his gall bladder removed.

He's not the only one I have heard this story from. Throughout all of my "how did you lose your gall bladder?" conversations with friends and strangers, it is a recurring theme: Loss of gall bladder, following greasy food binge, following strict lowfat or vegetarian diet.

Before I tell you why this happens, I will need to tell you some things you may not want to hear. Your body evolved to eat, digest, and process animal meats and fats. If your ancestors did not feast regularly on tasty animals, you would not be here to read this.

As a result of this evolution, you have a gall bladder. It is not a vestigial organ like the appendix. It has a purpose, and it needs regular exercise.

What happens when you run your body on a low-fat or strict vegetarian diet for a long period is that the gall bladder does not get a good workout. It is designed to handle heavy fat loads and it needs those on occasion to stay healthy. If there is no need for it to force out a heavy bile outflow, its contents will not circulate well, and the tendency for bile to crystallize and form stones within it will increase greatly.

In addition, the abundance of phytosterols (plant-based cholesterol) and lack of animal cholesterol creates a hormonal environment in your body which biases you towards decreased gall bladder activity and increased risk of gallstone formation (see chapter "Cholesterol" for specifics).

Then, one day, when that cheeseburger or bucket of fried chicken strikes and derails you from your steadfast vegetarian diet, your gall bladder will be ill-prepared to deal with the stones that have formed within it while it was collecting dust in that forgotten corner of your guts.

This is not to say that all vegetarians or low-fat dietarians will get gallstones-- it just increases your risk.

If and while you are on these diets, you should make sure to eat a fatty meal at least once a week. It need not contain animal fats (salads heavy on the olive oil will do the trick-- in addition the oil will help transfer the fat-soluble vitamins in the salad).

All moral issues aside, you really are missing out on good stuff your body legitimately needs if you skip out on the meat.

At least eat some eggs or milk. Those aren't cute and cuddly but they still taste good and contain animal fats.

# 11: Post-surgery Symptoms

If you have had your gall bladder removed and things are not quite right with your digestion, you may be experiencing the following problems.

**Postcholecystectomy Syndrome:**

Also known as PCS, this is a group of symptoms caused by changes in the bile flow due to the loss of the gall bladder. It affects roughly 15% of patients who have had their gall bladders removed. Fortunately the cause of PCS can be identified in 95% of patients.

PCS consists of two primary issues:

☐ Increased bile flow into the upper gastrointestinal (GI) tract, causing esophagitis and gastritis. This is similar to acid reflux.

☐ Increased bile flow into the lower GI tract causing diarrhea and colicky lower abdominal pain or discomfort.

What causes PCS is that once the gall bladder is removed, the circulation of bile in the entire GI system is altered. Bile output during fasting (when you are not eating) is higher because the gall bladder is no longer present to store it. Therefore it has nowhere to go but into your intestine, where it is introduced without other things to counteract it (such as stomach acid, food, etc). It can then cause irritation, laxative effects, and spasms of the GI tract and colon. Or it can back up into your stomach and cause mayhem there as well.

In a study done on PCS by Dr. R Peterli, a 65% majority of patients had no symptoms. However 28% had mild symptoms, 5% had moderate symptoms, and 2% had severe symptoms. The same study also found that the vast majority of symptoms were caused by a bile system functional disorder (such as irritable sphincter) at 26%. The other contending causes were minor: peptic disease at 4%, wound pain 2.4%, stones 1%, subhepatic fluid 0.8%, and incisional hernia at 0.4%.[1]

Getting a proper workup for PCS should include the following laboratory tests. Many of these tests are common, affordable, and can be done by any blood testing laboratory worldwide:

☐ **A CBC (Complete Blood Count)** screen to check for any disease or infections.

☐ **Basic Metabolic Panel (BMP)** contains checks for a broad range of nutritional items.

☐ **Amylase screen** to check for pancreatic disease.

☐ **Hepatic Function Panel (HFP)** to check the status of your liver function (or lack thereof).

☐ **Prothrombin Time (PT)** which is a test of blood's clotting abilities (coagulation), an indicator of Vitamin K status and a way to check for possible liver damage.

1    PeterliR,MerkiL,SchuppisserJP,AckermannC,HerzogU,TondelliP. [Postcholecystectomycomplaints one year after laparoscopic cholecystectomy. Results of a prospective study of 253 patients]. *Chirurg*. Jan 1998;69(1):55-60. [Medline].

*PCS imaging tests may include:*

☐ Barium swallow

☐ Upper GI and small bowel follow-through (SBFT) to check for esophagitis or gastroesophageal reflux disease (GERD/acid reflux) and peptic ulcer disease (PUD).

☐ Esophagastroduodenoscopy (EGD) which can replace the above battery of imaging tests.

☐ A CT scan if you are unable to do the above tests.

☐ Ultrasound to check the dilation of the common bile duct.

☐ An ERCP, or cholangiogram (or its long name Endoscopic Retrograde Cholangio-Pancreatography) described in the "Indentifying Gallstones" section above. This is described as being, hands-down, the best method for identifying causes of PCS, as it can identify post-surgical problems, hidden stones or blockages, and witness firsthand the activity and dilation of the bile ducts and the proper or improper behavior of the Sphincter of Oddi. In addition to being an excellent diagnostic tool can be used to treat many potential problems found during the exploratory procedure.

*Treating PCS:*

Treatments can be medical or surgical. It may be as simple as adding bulking agents such as fiber to the diet. Antispasmodics or sedatives may also help.

Cholestyramine has proven excellent in treating diarrhea associated with PCS as well as Habba Syndrome (see below). Antacids, histamine blockers, H-2 receptor blockers or proton pump inhibitors such as Pepcid, Zantac, and Prilosec, can help with reflux symptoms. Lovastatin also shows promising results, however statins are potentially dangerous for long term use.

In most cases surgery is not needed. And, as always, surgery should be considered only as a last resort. The ERCP procedure (described above) can assess whether or not a surgical procedure would be beneficial or even necessary. If there is, for example, problematic scarring, adhesions, or other damage to the bile ducts as a result of the cholecystectomy, it may be necessary to surgically remove scar tissue or perform a biliary bypass. In cases of sphincter damage or scarification, it may be necessary to remove the sphincter entirely.

## Habba Syndrome:

Habba Syndrome, named for Dr. Saad Habba, its discoverer, is often misdiagnosed as IBS. Most often it results in chronic and urgent watery diarrhea, especially after meals. Where it differs from IBS is that it is not caused by ulcers in the digestive tract; it is caused by malabsorption of bile salts in the small intestine. IBS is normally accompanied by cramping; Habba Syndrome is not. People attempting to treat Habba Syndrome with drugs meant for IBS will not see positive results.

The characteristics of IBS vs. Habba Syndrome are as follows:

| IBS | Habba Syndrome |
| --- | --- |
| Abdominal pain/cramps. | No abdominal pain. |
| Alternating bowel habits: both constipation and diarrhea. | Always post-prandial (after eating) diarrhea. |
| No change with fasting. | Improves with fasting. |
| Normal gall bladder function. | Poor gall bladder function. |
| Good response to antispasmodic drugs. | Poor response to antispasmodics. |
| Unpredictable response to bile acid resins. | Excellent response to bile acid resins. |

Diarrhea from Habba Syndrome may be difficult or impossible to control. Sufferers often commit "bathroom mapping" to their top priority in public places so they always know where to run when their symptoms appear.

While the syndrome has only been written about since 2000, it is believed that the cause is gall bladder dysfunction or bile salt malabsorption; some people who still have their gall bladders suffer from this syndrome. 1 in every 15 people who have their gall bladders removed also suffer from Habba Syndrome.

When bile salts are not reabsorbed in the end portion of the small intestine (ileum), they pass on to the large intestine and then attract water on a molecular level, which causes diarrhea. The bile salts themselves can also cause irritation in the large intestine and spasms of the colon.

Cholestyramine has proven an excellent medicine for treating the diarrhea for both Habba Syndrome and PCS. It is a resin which is mixed with water and taken orally, usually 30 minutes prior to meals. It is effective within 24-48 hours. Many patients, your author included, find that their lives have been miraculously restored with daily doses of Cholestyramine. This medicine is also sold under the name Questran, Questran Light (sugar-free), and Cholybar. Other bile acid sequestrants that do the same job are sold under the names Cholesevelam, Cholestagel, Welchol, Colestipol, and Colestid.

Cholestyramine works by binding up bile salts and rendering them inert. The inert compound is then passed in your excrement. The deactivated bile salts which then pass on to your large intestine can no longer attract water nor cause irritation, curing the urgent diarrhea.

Patients of Crohn's disease who have had their ileum surgically removed will suffer from bile salt malabsorption and therefore suffer the same symptoms as people with Habba Syndrome. Therefore it should come as no surprise that they are treated with Cholestyramine.

Since your body's bile supply is not being reabsorbed and recycled, cholesterol is then pulled from your bloodstream to supply bile production. This does have negative potential. Cholesterol is required by your body to repair cell walls, build sex hormones, and keep your brain and nervous system functioning properly. If you are not retaining an adequate supply on hand for your body to use because it is getting flushed down the toilet, the long term effects could be detrimental. For more information on deficiencies and malabsorption, read on to the next chapter.

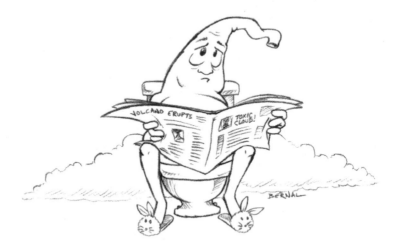

# 12: The Ugly Consequences of Malabsorption

When your body is no longer digesting properly, it is also not absorbing nutrients properly. The following things may result from a dysfunctional or removed gall bladder:

## Fat Soluble Vitamins and Deficiencies:

Some vitamins are only able to be absorbed if they ride along through the intestinal wall on the back of a fat molecule. These vitamins are A, D, E, and K. If the body has inadequate intake of these vitamins, some health problems can result. However, be aware that megadosing them is toxic and can lead to numerous health problems. They are easier to overdose (hypervitaminosis) than water-soluble vitamins as they are stored in the liver and fatty tissues of the body, eliminated much more slowly, and therefore remain in your system for a longer period of time.

Fat soluble vitamins are not destroyed during the cooking of the food that contains them.

# Vitamin A

Normal daily intake: 600-900 micrograms

Vitamin A consists of Retinol, Retinal, and four Carotenoids including Beta Carotene (a vitamin-A precursor). Its role is important in the production and development of bones and teeth, reproduction, cell division, gene expression, and the maintenance of mucous membranes.

**Sources of Vitamin A:** Mostly animal sources, including:

- Eggs
- Meat
- Milk/dairy products

**Sources of Beta Carotene:**

- Leafy greens
- Brightly colored vegetables (carrots, bell peppers)

**Vitamin A deficiency symptoms:**

- Night blindness: difficulty or inability to see in dimly lit places. It brings real meaning to the urban legend that eating carrots can help you see in the dark.
- Keratomalacia (dryness of the eye's cornea)

**Vitamin A overdose symptoms:**

- Birth defects
- Liver problems
- Reduced bone mineral density, osteoporosis, and coarse bone growths
- Skin discoloration, dryness, and peeling
- Hair loss
- Joint pain
- Headaches
- Fatigue
- Nausea
- Intercranial pressure (Idiopathic intracranial hypertension)
- Inflammation at the corners of the mouth (Angular cheilitis)

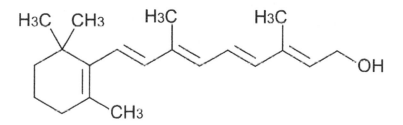

*Vitamin A*

# Vitamin D

Normal daily intake: 10 micrograms

Vitamin D, in addition to dietary intake, is manufactured by the body when it is exposed to sunlight. It is used to balance the body's use and absorption of calcium and phosphorous and plays a big role in bone production. The two most common forms of Vitamin D are D2 and D3.

**Sources of Vitamin D:**

- sunlight on your skin
- cheese
- butter and margarine
- fish

**Vitamin D deficiency symptoms:**

- Seasonal Affective Disorder (SAD), a form of depression otherwise known as the "Winter Blues." Sunscreen with a level of protection as low as SPF-8 can inhibit more than 95% of vitamin D production in the skin.

- Rickets (deformity of long bones, softening and thinning of bones)

- Osteoporosis

- Osteomalacia (thinning of the bones)

**Vitamin D overdose symptoms:**

- Dehydration
- Vomiting
- Decreased appetite (anorexia)
- Irritability
- Constipation
- Fatigue
- Hypercalcimia (elevated blood calcium levels)
- Hypertension

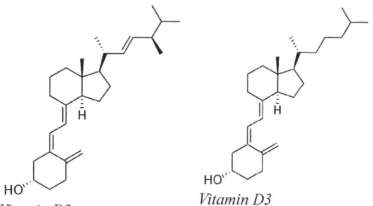

*Vitamin D2*

*Vitamin D3*

# Vitamin E

Normal daily intake: 10 milligrams

Vitamin E's main role is as an antioxidant, protecting blood cells and fatty acids from destruction by free radicals. Lack of vitamin E causes neurological problems stemming from poor nerve conduction. Vitamin E deficiency rarely occurs from a poor diet, but is seen often in people who cannot absorb dietary fat. That would be *us*.

**Sources of Vitamin E:**

- corn
- nuts
- olives
- avocado
- leafy greens
- vegetable oil
- wheat germ

**Vitamin E deficiency symptoms:**

- Neuromuscular dysfunction
- Spinocerebellar ataxia (progressive degradation of gait and coordination of hands, speech, eyes)
- Anemia
- Muscle weakness

- Degradation of the retina and eventual blindness

## Vitamin E overdose symptoms:
- Flushed skin
- Increased bleeding (Vitamin E is an anticoagulant)

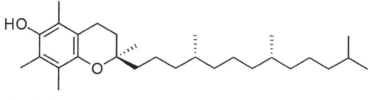

*Vitamin E*

# Vitamin K

Normal daily intake: 80 micrograms

Vitamin K is produced in our digestive system by friendly bacteria. It is also supplemented by what we eat. It acts primarily in blood clotting and bone health. People with digestive imbalances (such as diarrhea) which may cause lack of adequate intestinal bacteria, or improper populations of the proper intestinal bacteria (for example: us, with improper digestive function) are more prone to Vitamin K deficiencies.

**Sources of Vitamin K:**

- cabbage
- cauliflower
- broccoli
- beets
- spinach
- asparagus
- leafy greens

**Vitamin K deficiency symptoms:**

- Osteoporosis
- Coronary heart disease
- Anemia
- Easy bruising

- Bleeding gums
- Nosebleeds
- Heavy menstrual bleeding

**Vitamin K overdose symptoms:**

- Skin rash
- Diarrhea
- Nausea
- Vomiting
- Anemia
- Liver damage

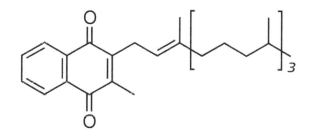

*Vitamin K1*

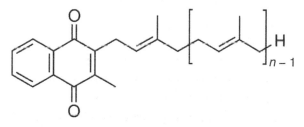

*Vitamin K2*

# 13: Our Friend Cholesterol

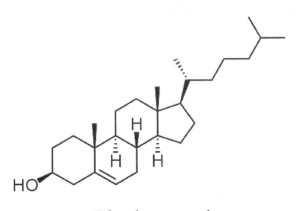

## Cholesterol

Normal daily intake: 300 milligrams

Cholesterol gets a lot of bad press but it is absolutely, essentially vital to life as we know it. Cholesterol is responsible for the construction, permeability, and fluidity of cell membranes, the production of bile, and the synthesis of hormones and Vitamin D. It is the fuel that powers your brain, and without it your body would cease to function at all. You would, quite literally, fall apart.

Cholesterol comes into play both by dietary intake, and by synthesis. As it is a compound required for cellular metabolism on many levels, your liver and other glands (aka lymphatic system) will manufacture it from component parts when necessary. If your body needs cholesterol and it cannot draw from supplies available in the bloodstream (ie: dietary intake) it will cannibalize it from other parts of your body. And if you cannot get an adequate supply from autocannibalism, your body will start shutting down other important but less-vital processes, such as hormone production. This is why human beings simply cannot survive without it, as militant as they may be about their health and diet.

Heart disease is the leading cause of death in the USA. There is a strong link to cholesterol and heart disease-- after all, heart disease would not be possible without cholesterol. But the cause and effect of heart disease are not as simple as that-- cholesterol is just one actor in a complex plot, and sticking it with the entire blame is wrong. We will explain this in detail as we explore the other fat actors and how they conspire to aid in your health, or your demise.

Let us now dispel some of the myths and ignorance surrounding cholesterol...

When you hear about "good" and "bad" cholesterol, those names refer not to cholesterol specifically, but its delivery mechanism. You see, cholesterol is always cholesterol-- it is neither good nor bad, it is simply the equivalent of a manufactured tool kit for your cells, most of it forged in the factory of your liver, and then shipped off to the far-flung provinces of your body. It cannot travel on its own, however. It needs a transport vehicle.

There are several vehicles it may travel in, and some of them are more "reliable" than others. It is this vehicle, not the cholesterol itself, which determines the "goodness" or "badness." This improper naming and labeling is unfortunate, because it causes people to make poor decisions regarding their diet and cut out cholesterol

97

when they need it.

Cholesterol, as a type of fat, is not water soluble, and therefore not blood-soluble. In order to make its way around your body it must travel inside a Lipoprotein molecule. The lipoprotein is like a truck, and the cholesterol its cargo. The liver is the central freight station in your body.

These lipoprotein trucks have five different sizes, in order from largest to smallest:

**Chylomicrons**: These large heavy-duty lipoprotein molecules are responsible for transporting fats, fatty acids, and dietary cholesterol from the intestines to the liver. They are manufactured 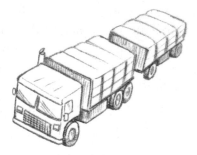 by the intestine, used to do their job, and then are broken down by the liver in order to make other lipoprotein formations...

**VLDL** (Very Low Density Lipoprotein): These are the stock lipopritein tucks manufactured by the liver. They transport cholesterol synthesized in the liver to other cells in the body. As they become used, they degrade into IDLs and eventually LDLs.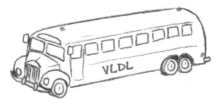

**IDL** (Intermediate Density Lipoprotein): These are degraded VLDL molecules, old trucks that have seen better days. They can still do their job, but eventually when they make their way back to the liver, they will be rehabilitated into LDLs.

**LDL (**Low Density Lipoprotein): These are the work-horses of cholesterol delivery. Their job is to transport cholesterol from the liver to other cells. Primarily, they travel the outgoing routes from the liver to other cells, however they can sometimes be used to pull cholesterol from other tissues and carry it back to the liver.

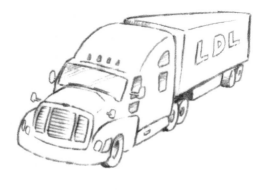

**HDL** (High Density Lipoprotein): These smaller freight vehicles are called out on pick-up duty to collect cholesterol from the body's tissues and bring them to the liver or other steroid-producing organs such as the testes, ovaries, and adrenal glands.

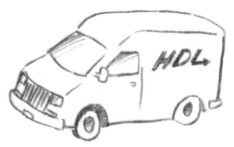

Both the type of the truck and the destination cells will affect the transportation of the cholesterol passenger. When a cell requires cholesterol, or desires to ship out extra cholesterol, it will open a "parking space" on its cell membrane, called a receptor.

These receptor parking spaces are built to accommodate specific types of lipoprotein vehicles. Should one of these specific trucks be driving by when the space opens up, it will park.

Cells looking to shed cholesterol will mainly open parking spaces for HDL, and cells needing more cholesterol will open spaces for LDL. It is possible for cells offloading surplus cholesterol to flag down LDL trucks in a process called "reverse cholesterol transport".

The various vehicles not only move cholesterol from cell to cell; they can meet mid-route and exchange cargo and spare parts. Some of this exchange between IDL and HDL results in the streamlining of IDL into LDL.

The delivery vehicles we are most concerned about are HDL and LDL.

HDL helps fight against oxidation, inflammation, arterial plaque, and platelet buildup, which are the sources of heart disease. Current medical recommendations are that 30% of your blood-cholesterol content be HDL.

Men are geneticallly predisposed to have much lower levels of HDL in their bloodstream than women, which explains why men are much more likely to suffer from heart disease than women.

The LDL vehicles are larger than HDL, their surfaces are not as smooth, and they are not as maneuverable. LDL is like the clunky old jalopy counterpart to the svelte shape of HDL.

LDL molecules cause problems when they are called to deliver healing cholesterol to inflamed tissues; arterial walls, in particular. After they have parked and dropped off their cargo, LDL molecules have a tendency to get jammed in the "parking space," tangled in glycoproteins within the cell wall of arterial tissue.

To make matters worse, the improperly-parked truck then catches the attention of white blood cells, which, acting like meter-maids booting a car, surround and engulf the LDL molecule and then harden in place.

Furthermore, the poor cell which had called for help in reducing its inflammation now has extra junk stuck to it which causes even *more* inflammation! This process is what causes the buildup of arterial plaque, which grows into arterial blockage, which then causes heart attacks and strokes.

## A Day In the Life of Cholesterol

Cholesterol first comes into your diet in the form of human breast milk. Well, it was being transferred to you from your mother's blood supply long before that, but in order to supply your rapidly-developing brain and body after you are born, you need a strong source of cholesterol, and you will find it in mother's milk.

Once you are old enough to ingest solid foods, your main dietary cholesterol intake arrives in the form of meat, eggs, cheese, and seafood. It is possible to gain dietary cholesterol from plants in the form of phytosterols (plant oils) but they occur in significantly smaller volumes in vegetable format. We'll come back to phytosterols in a

101

bit.

When you eat foods containing cholesterol, it is sequestered inside bile micelles during digestion. The lipids are then broken down by lipase and absorbed by your intestinal epithelial cells. These cells then reassemble and push these lipids out the other side into chylomicron transport trucks to carry them to the liver, via the bloodstream, for processing.

Your liver is the largest factory in your body for the production of cholesterol and hormones. It also builds the various VLDL, LDL, and HDL lipoprotein vehicles responsible for moving cholesterol molecules to and from the various cells in your body.

To increase your HDL levels, it is recommended that you increase your dietary intake of Omega-3 and Omega-6 fatty acids. We'll get to describing fatty acids and what they do in the next chapter.

The human body needs to ingest an average of 300mg of cholesterol daily (the equivalent of 2 egg yolks) for proper maintenance. That is in addition to the 3000mg (3 grams) it synthesizes daily. If you are more active, for example bodybuilding or undergoing strenuous physical work or exercise, your body will need more in order to keep your tissues repaired and keep up with your higher metabolism.

Most of the cholesterol activity in your body involves synthesis and recycling. 20-25% of cholesterol synthesis occurs in the liver. The remainder is done in the intestines, adrenal glands, and reproductive organs.

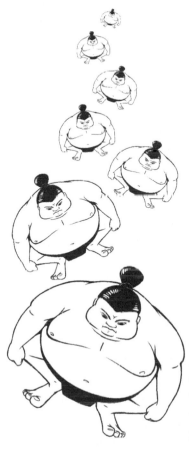

Various nutrients and chemical components in the body are taken up by these organs and assembled into cholesterol for use wherever it is needed. Throughout all this chemical shredding and reassembly, a portion of your cholesterol "bank balance" is lost, and that missing balance must be re-deposited via your dietary intake.

Cholesterol is lost or consumed simply because it is a building block of many things: it is used to build and patch cell membranes, it is converted into hormones, or vitamins, or excreted in the form of bile (5% of which, on average, is not reabsorbed). Your body's cells divide and reproduce, or die, or are shed: 40-50,000 skin cells per day for example. Each cell division needs more cholesterol to supply its cell membranes, and each shed cell takes with it a bit of that cell membrane, and therefore cholesterol.

If you do not get your 300mg of daily cholesterol from your diet, this means that your body must pull it from other sources. As it runs out of blood-borne nutrients, your body will slow down or shut off the production of things requiring cholesterol:

103

- Sex hormones like estradiol, testosterone, and progesterone, aldosterone, retinoic acid, and vitamin D

- Cortisol, which is responsible for blood sugar regulation and immune defenses

- Aldosterone, which regulates cellular hydration, salts, and kidney function

Furthermore, if the body continues to starve for fresh sources of cholesterol, it will begin to disassemble and cannibalize its own living cells. This is obviously not the situation you want to be in.

To make a long story short, your body needs a minimum "bank balance" of cholesterol to stay healthy. What you should remember is that the average Joe needs 300mg of cholesterol each day to provide for the fact that he has living animal tissue that needs its cell membranes replenished, and if he does not supply that amount he will begin to decay on a cellular level and eventually die.

Knowing all this, you may find it extremely frustrating to dig through ignorant misinformation in books and on the internet, especially if it is being spread by organizations like the American Heart Association, whose website says, "Typically the body makes all the cholesterol it needs, so people don't need to consume it."[2] If that doesn't make you want to jump in front of a bus, I don't know what will. No wonder the public can't get educated with the truth about fats and cholesterol-- the very places they look to for information are incorrect!!!

---

2   http://www.americanheart.org/presenter.jhtml?identifier=4488

## The Perfect Storm of Heart Disease

Heart Disease is the leading cause of death in the USA. Initially, and in some ways presently, a high level of LDL blood cholesterol was thought to be the primary cause.

Recent studies now point to the fact that high blood cholesterol has less to do with heart disease than does the actual cause of the arterial plaque buildup, which is *inflammation*. Inflammation of the tissues is caused by poor nutrition, elevated blood sugar, and high blood pressure (which is a prime result of the previous two).

Improper diets, the kind that cause tissue inflammation, will almost always cause high levels of LDL from the intake of trans-fats and hydrogenated fats. The body has to transport the overabundance of fats it is taking in, and it can only do it with chylomicrons which become LDL. Because the LDL is in ample supply, it will readily be used to convey cholesterol to the cells for repair, and increase the odds of getting stuck in the cell wall.

Then, as you've read, the white blood cells come by to patch over the rough spot, they harden in place, and arterial plaque forms. The arterial plaque has a tendency to cause more inflammation, which calls for more lipoprotein trucks to transport more cholesterol to fix the cell walls. More trucks are sent out, and more get stuck. The cycle repeats until the arteries are hardened and blocked, and the heart tissues cannot get enough blood flow to survive.

## Are you getting enough Cholesterol?

When in doubt, it is always better to have too much cholesterol than too little. Too little cholesterol is a condition called Hypocholesterolemia. This condition occurs when the body in question can no longer provide adequate cholesterol to support its cell membranes. Cellular metabolism grinds to a halt, and bad things happen. Hypocholesterolemia can be responsible for:

- Depression
- Hormonal shortages
- Loss of sex drive
- Cancer
- Cerebral Hemorrhage
- Death

Possible causes of Hypocholesterolemia:

- Statins (cholesterol-lowering medications)
- Hyperthyroidism (overactive thyroid gland)
- Liver disease
- Malabsorption (often caused by Coeliac Disease)
- Malnutrition
- Genetic predisposition (such as abetalipoproteinemia or hypobetalipoproteinemia). Jews get stuck with a higher risk of abetalipoproteinemia.
- Manganese deficiency
- Leukemia

## Are you getting too much cholesterol?

The flip-side of Hypocholesterolemia is Hypercholesterolemia. The Hyper part refers, simply, to "too much." Too much blood cholesterol could be caused by a number of things, mostly diet and genetic predisposition. Diet is easy to change, but genetics you are for life. Fortunately there are medications which can help you if diet alone cannot.

*Hypercholesterolemia can cause:*

☐ Plaque formation in the arteries

☐ Stenosis (narrowing) of the arteries due to blockage

☐ Death, from stroke or heart attack caused by the previous problems.

☐ Yellowish patches near the eyelids, caused by the formation of cholesterol deposits (aka Xanthelasma palpebrarum)

**Phytosterols and why they may not be good for you:**

As if you needed more things to worry about outside of HDL and LDL... Let's revisit phytosterols, the vegetarian brand of cholesterol.

Phytosterols, also called "plant sterols" are steroid alcohols, and differ slightly from animal cholesterol in their structure.

Phytosterols, when being absorbed, will actually "cut in line" to get into you first, and block the absorption of animal cholesterol. Even if there is an equal amount of both in your diet, the phytosterols will crowd out the channels that the cholesterol would use to enter your body, blocking their absorption. Not only does this block absorption of cholesterol introduced dietarily, it blocks reabsorption of bile. This is why some people eat plants high in phytosterols to reduce their blood cholesterol level-- it does work, in the same overall process as ingesting a pharmaceutical bile sequestrant.

What nobody tells you, or what they don't know, or what they definitely don't want you to hear is the following...

Animal cholesterol, chemically, is an unspecialized platform which will someday be a hormone. It isn't a hormone yet, nor is it sensed as one, until its molecular structure has been altered by your liver or glands with the addition of other molecular components.

Phytosterols, in contrast, arrive as cholesterol with extra hormonal tags already attached to them. The phytosterol Beta-sitosterol is the primary "precursor" phytosterol that many subsequent phytosterols originate from. It is also the worst for you. Beta-sitosterol, defined, is a plant-derived estrogen.

Beta-sitosterol causes nausea, diarrhea, gas, erectile dysfunction[3], and has negative side-effects inhibiting the production of the male hormones testosterone and dihydrotestosterone.[4] It is found in avocado, cashews, corn oil, pecans, pumpkin seeds, rice bran, saw palmetto, soybeans, and wheat germ.

Phytosterols in general are currently undergoing controversy; their previous reputation for good is turning out to be hype now that the long-term effects are being discovered. It is indesputable that phytosterols reduce blood cholesterol, but studies are beginning to show that they do more harm than good.[5]

Within the Stigmasterol group of phytosterols, for example, is also the precursor to the hormone progesterone. Even if these hormonal precursors may not get the finishing touches put on them to be molecularly perfect, many have the ability to interact with and trigger receptors in the body built to connect with the finished hormones. These unwanted interactions can cause crossed hormonal signals.

---

3   Kristi Monson, PharmD; Arthur Schoenstadt, MD (February 2008).
4   Selvarajah D, Gandhi R, Emery CJ, Tesfaye S. (October 2009). "Randomized placebo-controlled double-blind clinical trial of cannabis-based medicinal product (Sativex) in painful diabetic neuropathy: depression is a major confounding factor". *Diabetes Care* **161** (1): 33.
5   Weingartner, O.; Bohm, M.; Laufs, U. (2008). "Controversial role of plant sterol esters in the management of hypercholesterolaemia". European Heart Journal 30 (4): 404–9.

*With a diet heavy in phytosterols you will:*

- ☐ Reduce absorption of cholesterol
- ☐ Reduce reabsorption of bile
- ☐ Therefore lowering your blood cholesterol, resulting in...
- ☐ Reduction in the synthesis of vitamin D, estradiol, testosterone, aldosterol, and progesterone.
- ☐ An overabundance of leftover estrogen and progesterone precursors, resulting in...
- ☐ Lowered levels of estradiol and testosterone, amid plenty of estrogen and progesterone, which can result in a laundry list of unsavory things...

*Side effects of elevated progesterone levels:*

- ☐ Progesterone is used as hormone therapy for male-to-female sex changes. It will actually cause men to develop female breasts. It will also alter male behavior to bend towards the female behavior spectrum. Summed up, men will become physically and mentally more feminine.
- ☐ Increased risk of blood clots, heart attacks, and stroke.
- ☐ Increased risk of breast cancer.
- ☐ Cramps, headaches, constipation, flatulence.
- ☐ Nervousness, emotional instability, depression, mood swings, hot flashes, insomnia, loss of short term memory.
- ☐ Decreased sex drive, erectile dysfunction.

☐ And last, but not least: **Reduced gall bladder activity**!!! Yes, progesterone has a role to play in telling your gall bladder to be lazy.

*Side effects of elevated estrogen levels:*

☐ Estrogen is the primary female sex hormone, whose job it is, among other things, to promote secondary female sex characteristics, such as body structure. It will, like progesterone, have a feminizing effect on men both mentally and physically.

☐ Estrogen **reduces bowel motility** and **increases cholesterol concentration in bile**, meaning that it increases the risk of gallstones. Couple this with reduced gall bladder activity from extra progesterone, and you are bound to have problems.

☐ Reduction in muscle mass.

☐ Increase in body fat storage.

☐ Increase blood levels of HDL and decrease blood levels of LDL (this is why men usually have lower HDL levels)

## Controlling cholesterol problems

There are only three solutions that are 100% guaranteed to bring a halt to the absorption of LDL. Those solutions are to:

1. Stop eating.

2. Remove your liver.

3. Die.

Obviously, death has very unpleasant and undesirable side effects: coldness of skin, rigor mortis, "respiratory difficulty," body odor, etc.

And, unfortunately, option 1 and 2 both lead to option 3. It may be impossible to eliminate all LDL from your diet but it is EASY to reduce it to low levels.

It is therefore important that we use our brains (which run on cholesterol, by the way!) and explore other methods, which are not 100% effective but worth a try:

1. The natural way, the best way, and the cheapest way, which is done by learning what is in the foods you eat, and trying to reduce your intake of the bad stuff. Dietary control can work wonders, and unless you have a serious medical condition, it is the most effective and least destructive to your body.

2. Bile acid sequestrants, such as Cholestyramine. These are taken orally, usually as a powder mixed with water, and will bind to bile in the digestive tract, making it impossible to reabsorb. This process will cause the body to re-stock bile by pulling cholesterol out of the blood supply, thereby reducing your blood cholesterol levels. Bile acid

113

sequestrants to not discriminate in the type of lipoproteins they help remove; that is up to the liver to decide. Bile acid sequestrants are the lowest-impact method of reducing blood cholesterol levels via medication.

3. Dietary supplementation with phytosterols. So long as you know that this can potentially cause you some major issues long-term, it is a relatively low-impact solution for the short-term. You do not need to go on a strict vegetarian diet to benefit from their effect, as they will block out the absorption of animal cholesterol. But do know the side effects and downsides-- study continues on whether or not the benefit is worth the hazard.

4. Statins, such as Lovostatin, are cholesterol inhibitors that work to block synthesis of cholesterol in the liver. They will reduce manufacture of LDL but they will not increase HDL. To get proper cholesterol balance you will still need to alter your diet for higher HDL production, even with the assistance of statins. Statins in combination with a vegetarian diet is a recipe for disaster.

## Where do Lipoproteins and Cholesterol come from, and how can I increase my HDL levels?

Cholesterol enters your body dietarily. When you eat foods containing cholesterol, it is sequestered with other fats inside bile micelles during digestion. The fats are then absorbed by your intestinal epithelial cells. These cells then build chylomicron transport trucks to carry the fat and cholesterol to the liver for processing, and push them out into the bloodstream.

The primary origin of both LDL and HDL is your liver. It is the largest factory in your body for the production of cholesterol and hormones. It also builds and restructures the lipoprotein vehicles responsible for moving cholesterol molecules to and from the cells which need them. Your liver makes HDL as well as LDL and all the others.

To increase your HDL levels, it is recommended that you increase your dietary intake of:

- Omega-3 fatty acids
- Omega-6 fatty acids
- monounsaturated, polyunsaturated, and saturated fatty acids

Quitting smoking has also been proven to increase HDL levels.

To decrease your LDL levels, you should:

- eliminate intake of trans fats

- reduce intake of sugars and refined grain products like bread and corn syrup
- lose weight
- increase soluble fiber in the diet (oats, barley, kidney beans, prunes, apples and pears)
- increase intake of polyunsaturated fatty acids, found commonly in nuts of all kinds

# 14: Fatty Acids

A fatty acid, defined in layman's terms, is a hydrocarbon molecule with a long, unbranched tail or "chain" of carbon atoms. These carbon tail atoms typically have two hydrogen atoms stuck to them, one on each side along the tail. Fatty acids are components of triglycerides (remember our explanation of what remains of lipids after the Lipase Samura chops them up) and phospholipids, which are what cell walls are constructed of.

While your body can manufacture some fatty acids, it cannot supply adequate amounts to keep you running; if it did, we would never have to eat.

Fatty acids are important in your diet because they are metabolized by your cells' mitochondria into ATP, the fuel of all cellular life. Most cells have a choice between glucose or fatty acids, and are capable of converting them both into ATP. Your heart and skeletal muscles, however, having more mitochondria, prefer to metabolize fatty acids to get their ATP.

Fatty acids come in many shapes and sizes, but what differentiates them from each other is typically the number of carbon atoms in their tail, and whether they are saturated or unsaturated.

### Size does matter:

Short chain fatty acids have tails of fewer than 6 carbon atoms. Medium Chain fatty acids have 6 to 12, Long Chain fatty acids have 13 to 21, and Very Long Chain fatty acids have 22 and higher. Most naturally occurring fatty acids have even numbers of carbon atoms.

Generally speaking, short and medium chain fatty acids are considered good for you as they are easier to absorb and metabolize. They can be absorbed directly into the intestine and sent straight into your bloodstream. Hence they are an instant and healthy source of cellular energy.

While long-chain Omega-3 and Omega-6 fatty acids are very good for you, some long chain fatty acids can be hazardous because they cannot be directly absorbed into the intestine, and they require the intestinal cells to produce a chylomicron transport to move them when they are converted into a triglyceride on the other side of the epithelial wall. Long chain fatty acids, especially from trans fats, can indeed raise your LDL cholesterol levels.

### Unsaturated or monounsaturated:

Whether the fatty acids are saturated or not is defined by how they bind to hyrdogen, which is determined by the occurrence of double-carbon bonds in the molecule's tail. Unsaturated fatty acids have one or more double carbon bonds. Monounsaturated refers to a molecule with only one double-carbon bond. This double-carbon bond not only prevents hydrogen molecules from binding to it, but it can also cause a bend in the shape of the molecule.

Naturally-occurring unsaturated fatty acids have what is called a "cis" configuration in the double carbon bond, which creates the bend in the tail. These bends have mechanical effects on how they fit together, and what they can and cannot be used for. The shape of the fatty acids also affects their melting points and ability to oxidize. Most unsaturated fats are liquid at room temperature, and go rancid quickly via the process of oxidation.

### *Polyunsaturated:*

A polyunsaturated fatty acid is a molecule which contains more than one double-carbon bond. Omega-3 and Omega-6 are examples of polyunsaturated fatty acids.

Why 3 and 6? The number refers to the position of the last double-carbon bond, counted from the end of the chain. For example, see ALA, an Omega-3:

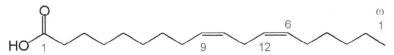

If you count back from the end on the right side of the diagram, there are 2 "zigs" of single carbon, and the third "zag" is a double-carbon bond. It being the last in the chain and on the third spot from the end, makes it an Omega-3. Similar naming rules apply for Linoleic Acid, an Omega-6, where the final double-carbon bond occurs in spot 6 from the end:

### *Saturated:*

Saturated fatty acids are those without double carbon bonds, allowing the full tail of the molecule to be available for hydrogen bonds (and therefore, saturated, with hydrogen). Saturated fatty acids are less prone to oxidation and rancidity.

For this reason, saturated fats are preferred in cooking, baking, and modern processed food because they are more solid and stable at room temperature, and have a longer shelf life.

### Hydrogenation and trans fats:

The industrial process of hydrogenation is used to "reinforce" unsaturated fats, by forcing extra hydrogen into the molecule. This chemical forcing flips over the double-carbon link in the chain, straightening out the molecule, and allowing more hydrogen to move in and stick, making the molecule less reactive with oxygen and therefore longer-lasting. Such a flipped double-carbon link is called a "trans" configuration and is where the term "trans fat" comes from.

The specific mechanism by which trans fats cause you damage is not entirely known yet, but it is believed that Lipase cannot understand how to slice a molecule with a trans carbon bond and is therefore ineffective in dealing with breakdown of trans fats. This allows the trans fat to spend more time within the bloodstream where it will be more prone to stick in arterial walls and aid in plaque buildup.

What is known is that diets with a high level of trans fat put the eater at significantly higher risk of coronary heart disease, raise levels of LDL, and reduce levels of HDL. There is also evidence that trans fats increase risk of Alzheimer's disease, cancer, diabetes, liver dysfunction, depression, infertility, and obviously obesity.

### *Essential Fatty Acids (EFAs):*

Essential fatty acids cannot be manufactured or assembled from other components by your body, and thus must enter you via dietary intake. What designates a fatty acid as "essential" is the placement of a double-carbon bond after the 9th and 10th link in the chain. The human body is simply incapable of making this type of molecule.

Fortunately other creatures both animal and venetable *are* capable, and we can eat them in order to supply ourselves with their sophisticated fatty acids.

The two truly essential fatty acids which we cannot be without are known as LA (Linoleic Acid) and ALA (Alpha-Linoleic Acid). These EFAs are readily available in plant oils, which is where we get them from.

Other important fatty acids, while not quite essential, are Gamma-Linoleic Acid (an Omega-6), Lauric Acid, and Palmitoleic Acid. Others you may hear about are EPA (eicosapentaenoic acid) and DHA (docosahexaenoic acid), which are found in fish oil tablets. The human body does have the ability to produce EPA and DHA in limited quantities, but it fares much better if these are provided to it by dietary intake. Hence the tablets' popularity.

### Sources of short chain fatty acids:

☐ Dietary fiber fermented in your colon.

☐ Milk fat: goats, sheep, cows.

☐ Coconut oil.

### Sources of medium chain fatty acids:

☐ Milk fat: horse

☐ Coconut oil

☐ Palm kernel oil

### Sources of Omega-3 and Omega-6 long chain fatty acids:

☐ Fish, fish oil, krill, and certain shellfish like mussels.

☐ Oil seeds such as flax, hemp, chia, purslane.

☐ Nuts: walnuts, pecans, hazelnuts, butternuts.

☐ Eggs.

☐ Meat: grassfed beef has twice as much as grain-fed.

☐ Algae such as Crypthecodinium cohnii and Schizochytrium for those of you with vegan tendencies.

# 15: What Finally Worked for Me

It took several years of experimentation and research for me to find my particular dietary balance. My metabolic panels came back with results displaying perfect health. I had checked several ways for Coeliac Disease, all tests negative. No apparent food allergies, and according to all these tests I should have no problems whatsoever.

Bile supplementation did not work for me. Cholestyramine did help quite a bit, however, initially calming the urgency and unpredictability of my explosive bowels. I did not want to keep using it forever, but it did give me some comfortable refuge during my research.

The thing that had the biggest effect, believe it or not, was going on a low-gluten diet. Despite the fact that I do not have Coeliac Disease, it made a significant change. I no longer had bowel urgency after eating, and all the symptoms of Habba Syndrome disappeared.

It took about 10 days for the changes to be noticeable but it worked. I also lost 20 lbs, feel better, and have more energy. My poop is still not 100% dense and perfect but it's not blasting out of me like hot lava anymore. Regaining the freedom to poop when and where you wish to poop makes a big improvement in your overall quality of life, let me tell you! More experimentation will be required to tweak it to that final level of perfection but I have definitely reached a state where my mind and thoughts are no longer constantly occupied by my bowel movements. Liberty!

The only explanation I can think of is that I have some sort of intolerance but not an official allergy, and it caused intestinal degradation and atrophy. Similar to Coeliac Disease but not Coeliac Disease.

The dietary rules I use are a sort of cross between Paleo and Low-carb:

- ☐ No wheat, bread, or gluten-containing products unless you have no other choice.

- ☐ No soy.

- ☐ All meat and vegetables are fair game.

- ☐ I still eat rice and potatoes.

- ☐ Beer and liquor are OK, but wheat beers are off-limits.

If you really stop to think about it, there is so much wheat in the modern diet it is in every meal, if not every food item. It is hard to avoid.

Cutting out bread was hard at first. You crave it. You want it. You think about binging, jamming down a whole box of chocolate chip cookies. But then, one day, a couple of weeks later, you just lose the urge to deal with the stuff. It no longer tempts you, and the mere thought of it makes you lose your appetite.

Strange to wrap your head around but it's true. I never thought I would experience it, and always gave my wife, the ultimate Low-Carb/Paleo Nazi, a hard time about it. Turns out she was right.

Now this sort of thing might not work for

everyone, since everyone is different, but at least give it some thought. If all you have to lose is uncontrollable diarrhea, give it a try. You too might successfully liberate your intestines from their harsh indentured servitude!

# 16: All you can eat (and can't)

I'm not going to scold you into eating stuff you don't want to, but I am going to make some recommendations for stuff that might really help you out. For the most part you can eat an omnivorous diet; there are a few things that you should definitely stay away from, and some that you should definitely add. I'll keep it short and sweet.

*Avoid:*

☐ Processed foods heavy in grains or flour, especially wheat, hydrogenated oils, sugar and corn syrup. No more Twinkies or Little Debbie snack cakes. Unless you want to crap yourself.

☐ Large servings of pasta.

☐ Sugary soft drinks. If you are really addicted to soft drinks, try switching to diet ginger ale. It's better for you and the ginger provides a bowel-soothing side effect.

☐ Anything deep-fried.

☐ Breaded meat products, as they are usually deep-fried, contain low-grade meat and lots of fillers made of wheat and soy, and also tend to contain trans fats.

☐ Gravy. It just never ends well, trust me.

☐ Heavy use of salad dressing.

- Crisco, corn oil, or generic vegetable oil
- Margarine
- Prepared meals (TV Dinners, Le Menu, etc)
- Excessive consumption of caffeinated beverages
- Onion rings from Burger King (results worse than gravy)

## *Encourage:*

- Potatoes
- Butter
- Leafy greens
- Fish and other seafood
- Grass-fed beef
- Free-range chicken
- Well-treated pork
- Eggs from happy chickens
- Lean bacon
- Milk from any creature
- Fruits
- Nuts
- Vegetables
- Shrooms
- Carrots

- Beets
- Anything with dietary fiber
- Coconut oil, palm kernel oil, olive oil, sunflower oil (in order of better-for-you-ness)
- Ginger
- Yogurt
- Cheese

## Use sparingly:

- Rice
- Barley
- Oats
- Avocados (delicious and healthy but they get things moving if you know what I mean)
- Processed meats such as hot dogs, sausage, or pre-fab hamburgers

## Supplement:

- LA, ALA, EPA and DHA (Omega-3 and Omega-6 essential fatty acids/fish oil)
- Vitamins A, D, E, K
- Bile (if it helps)
- Pancreatin (if it helps)
- Lipase (if it helps)

131

# 17: Probably Useless Oddities

☐ Rats, deer, and horses do not have gall bladders.

☐ The average human produces about 24,000 liters of bile in their lifetime. That is enough to fill a large tanker truck!

# 18: Index

*Bile supplements and suppliers:*

*(Not by any means an exhaustive list)*

## Jarrow Formulas

*Web:* http://www.jarrow.com
*Email:* orders@jarrow.com
*Phone:* (310) 204-6936
*Products:* Bile Acid Factors, 333mg, 90 capsules.

## Supplement Facts

Serving Size 3 Capsules          Servings Per Container 30

| | Amount Per 3 Capsules | % DV |
|---|---|---|
| Total Bile Acids (from 1530 bovine/ovine bile concentrate) | 1000 mg | * |
| Conjugated Bile Acid (as glycocholic acid, taurocholic acid, glycodeoxycholic acid, taurodeoxycholic acid, glycochenodeoxycholic acid and taurochenodeoxycholic acid) | 945 mg | * |
| Unconjugated Bile Acid (as cholic acid and deoxycholic acid) | 55 mg | * |

* Daily Value not established.

## Nutricology

2300 North Loop Road
Alameda, CA 94502

*Web:* http://www.nutricology.com
*Phone:* (800) 545-9960
*Products:* Ox Bile, 125mg, 180 capsules. Ox Bile, 500mg, 100 capsules.

## Vital Nutrients

45 Kenneth Dooley Drive

Middletown, CT 06457

*Web:* http://www.vitalnutrients.net

*Phone:* (860) 638-3675

*Products:* Pancreatin & Ox Bile Extract

# Supplement Facts
serving size: 1 capsule

|  | amount per serving |
| --- | --- |
| Full Strength Pancreatin† providing: | 250mg* |
| Protease     55,700 USP units | |
| Amylase     61,250 USP units | |
| Lipase        8,875 USP units | |
| Ox Bile Extract | 100mg* |

* Daily Value not established

Other Ingredients: Vegetable Cellulose Capsule, Calcium Carbonate, and Leucine. † LACTOSE FREE

## Cholacol

Chiropractic Mindset Group

3200 North Hiawassee RD. Suite 3602

Orlando, FL 32868

*Web:* http://cholacol.com/

*Email:* Ron@cholacol.com

*Products:* Cholacol, 90 tablets (a blend of collinsonia root powder and bovine bile salts)

**Thorne Research**
P.O. Box 25
Dover, ID 83825
USA

*Web:* http://thorne.com/index.jsp
*Phone:* (800) 228-1966
*Products:* BioGest
**Betaine Hydrochloride** 480 mg.
**L-Glutamic Acid Hydrochloride** 480 mg.
**Pancreatin (Porcine)** 140 mg.
**Ox Bile Concentrate** 80 mg.
**Pepsin (Porcine)** 70 mg.

Please visit my website,
# www.gallbladderinfo.com
for articles, updates, resources, product referrals and
reviews, and new findings.

Made in the USA
Monee, IL
17 December 2020